Understanding Medicines Management for Nursing Students

Sara Miller McCune founded SAGE Publishing in 1965 to support the dissemination of usable knowledge and educate a global community. SAGE publishes more than 1000 journals and over 800 new books each year, spanning a wide range of subject areas. Our growing selection of library products includes archives, data, case studies and video. SAGE remains majority owned by our founder and after her lifetime will become owned by a charitable trust that secures the company's continued independence.

Los Angeles | London | New Delhi | Singapore | Washington DC | Melbourne

Understanding Medicines Management for Nursing Students

Paul Deslandes
Ben Pitcher
Simon Young

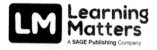

Learning Matters
A SAGE Publishing Company
1 Oliver's Yard
55 City Road
London EC1Y 1SP

SAGE Publications Inc.
2455 Teller Road
Thousand Oaks, California 91320

SAGE Publications India Pvt Ltd
B 1/I 1 Mohan Cooperative Industrial Area
Mathura Road
New Delhi 110 044

SAGE Publications Asia-Pacific Pte Ltd
3 Church Street
#10-04 Samsung Hub
Singapore 049483

First edition published in 2022

Editor: Laura Walmsley
Development editor: Sarah Turpie
Senior project editor: Chris Marke
Project management: River Editorial
Marketing manager: Ruslana Khatagova
Cover design: Sheila Tong
Typeset by: C&M Digitals (P) Ltd, Chennai, India

Library of Congress Control Number: 2022930473

British Library Cataloguing in Publication Data

A catalogue record for this book is available from the British Library

ISBN 978-1-5297-3082-1
ISBN 978-1-5297-3081-4 (pbk)

Contents

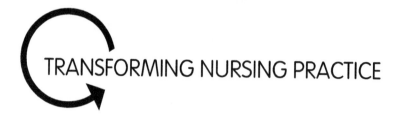

TRANSFORMING NURSING PRACTICE

Transforming Nursing Practice is a series tailor made for pre-registration student nurses. Each book in the series is:

 Clearly written and easy to read

Full of case studies and activities

✓ Mapped to the NMC Standards of proficiency for registered nurses

Focused on applying everyday nursing theory to practice

Each book addresses a core topic and has been carefully developed to be simple to use, quick to read and written in clear language.

An invaluable series of books that explicitly relates to the NMC standards. Each book covers a different topic that students need to explore in order to develop into a qualified nurse... I would recommend this series to all Pre-Registered nursing students whatever their field or year of study.

Many titles in the series are on our recommended reading list and for good reason - the content is up to date and easy to read. These are the books that actually get used beyond training and into your nursing career.

LINDA ROBSON,
Senior Lecturer at Edge Hill University

EMMA LYDON,
Adult Student Nursing

ABOUT THE SERIES EDITORS

DR MOOI STANDING is an Independent Academic Nursing Consultant (UK and international) responsible for the core knowledge, personal and professional learning skills titles. She has invaluable experience as an NMC Quality Assurance Reviewer of educational programmes, and as a Professional Regulator Panellist on the NMC Practice Committee. Mooi is also a Board member of Special Olympics Malaysia.

DR SANDRA WALKER is a Clinical Academic in Mental Health working between North Bristol Trust and Southern Health Trust. She is series editor for the mental health nursing titles. She is a Qualified Mental Health Nurse with a wide range of clinical experience spanning 30 years and spent several years working as a mental health lecturer at Southampton University.

BESTSELLING TEXTBOOKS

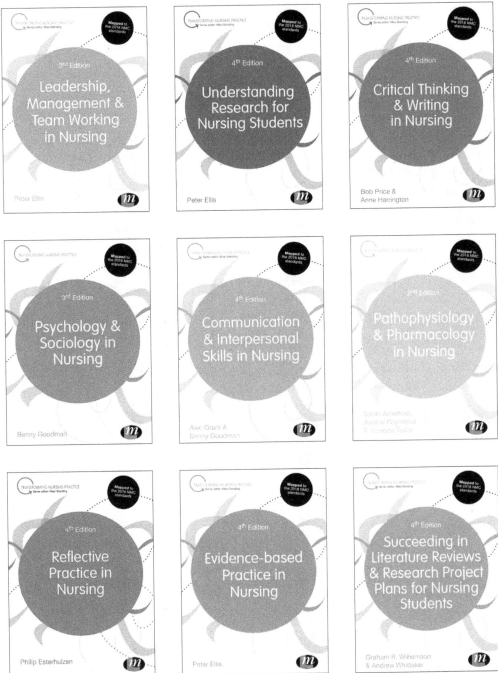

You can find a full list of textbooks in the *Transforming Nursing Practice* series at
uk.sagepub.com/TNP-series

About the authors

Paul Deslandes, BPharm, PhD, MRSB CBiol, is senior lecturer in medicines management and prescribing at the University of South Wales, and a pharmacist working at the All Wales Therapeutics and Toxicology Centre. Dr Deslandes studied pharmacy and went on to complete a PhD in neuropharmacology at the Welsh School of Pharmacy, Cardiff University. His research interests include the effectiveness and safety of medicines, in particular those used in the management of mental illness.

Ben Pitcher, BSc BN, MSc HEA is senior lecturer in life sciences and pharmacology at the University of South Wales, UK. After completing his first degree in pharmacology at Cardiff University, he went on to train as a nurse, after which he worked in critical care. He now teaches anatomy and physiology and medicines management to pre-registration and post-registration nurses and midwives, and manages the Independent Prescribing course. His teaching interest focuses on raising the level of medicines management and pharmacological knowledge across the profession.

Simon Young, BPharm, PhD, SFHEA is the Deputy Head of the School of Care Sciences at the University of South Wales. He is a registered pharmacist and pharmacist independent prescriber. Dr Young studied pharmacy and went on to complete a PhD in respiratory pharmacology at the Welsh School of Pharmacy, Cardiff University. His teaching interests include the application of pharmacological knowledge to medicines management in health and social care, developing prescribing competence and his research interests include the efficacy and safety of medicines and methods of developing numeracy competence in healthcare.

Acknowledgements

The authors would like to thank Donna Goddard, Sarah Turpie and Laura Walmsley, and all the other staff at SAGE who have helped us in the publication of this book. We would also like to acknowledge our families, who have been supportive as ever. Thank you to Jess Pitcher, who has been working on COVID-19 wards whilst Ben was at home typing away at his computer. Thank you to Dr Rhian Deslandes for discussions with Paul around some of the content.

Introduction

About this book

This book provides an introduction to some of the important aspects to consider when managing patients' medicines in clinical practice. We have tried to use a patient-centred approach, with case studies to reflect the contemporary perspective of medicines management. The book is principally aimed at undergraduate nursing students; however, it may also be of interest to students studying other healthcare-related courses.

Whilst this book has been written to support your knowledge and understanding of medicines management, it does not replace official procedures, guidance, frameworks or standards.

Book structure

The book is divided into eight chapters. Chapter 1 introduces you to two key reference sources that are used when managing medicines in the UK. These are the British National Formulary and the Summary of Product Characteristics for a medicine. You will use these references when completing exercises in the later chapters of the book. Chapter 2 introduces you to what we mean by a 'medicine' and how that is different to a 'drug'. It also explains how medicines are developed, and how this helps to ensure their quality, safety and efficacy. This chapter also introduces you to how drugs work, and to the way in which patients are able to access medicines.

Chapter 3 explores some of the legal and ethical aspects that need to be considered when managing medicines. These include the way in which medicines are classified and how this affects their management. It also considers how patient factors such as capacity and cultural and religious needs influence medicines use. Chapter 4 describes the ways in which medicines are administered to patients, and how the route of administration influences the medicine's formulation. It also considers the safe disposal of medicines after use.

Chapters 5 and 6 explore some of the adverse effects that medicines can have, and how physiological factors affect a patient's response to medicines. Chapter 7 explores some of the ways in which medicines can impact society more widely, and Chapter 8 considers how the evidence that supports use of a medicine can be interpreted (or in some cases misinterpreted).

Requirements for the NMC Standards of Proficiency for Registered Nurses

The Nursing and Midwifery Council (NMC) has established standards of proficiency to be met by applicants to different parts of the register, and these are the standards it considers necessary for safe and effective practice. This book is structured so that it will help you to understand and meet the proficiencies required for entry to the NMC register. The relevant proficiencies are presented at the start of each chapter so that you can clearly see which ones the chapter addresses. The proficiencies have been designed to be generic so apply to all fields of nursing and all care settings. This is because all nurses must be able to meet the needs of any person they encounter in their practice, regardless of their stage of life or health challenges, whether these are mental, physical, cognitive or behavioural.

This book includes the latest standards for 2018 onwards, taken from the *Future Nurse: Standards of proficiency for registered nurses* (NMC, 2018b).

Learning features

Learning from reading text is not always easy. Therefore, to provide variety and to assist with the development of independent learning skills and the application of theory to practice, this book contains activities, case studies, further reading, useful websites and other materials to enable you to participate in your own learning. You will need to develop your own study skills and 'learn how to learn' to get the best from the material. The book cannot provide all the answers, but instead provides a framework for your learning.

The activities in the book will in particular help you to make sense of, and learn about, the material being presented. Some activities ask you to reflect on aspects of practice, or your experience of it, or the people or situations you encounter. Reflection is an essential skill in nursing, and it helps you to understand the world around you and often to identify how things might be improved. Other activities will help you develop key graduate skills such as your ability to think critically about a topic in order to challenge received wisdom, or your ability to research a topic and find appropriate information and evidence, and to be able to make decisions using that evidence in situations that are often difficult and time-pressured. Communication is core to all nursing practice, and some activities will ask you to consider the way that you can use communication skills to support medicines management.

All the activities require you to take a break from reading the text, think through the issues presented and carry out some independent study, possibly using the internet. Where appropriate, there are sample answers presented at the end of each chapter, and these will help you to understand more fully your own reflections and independent study. Remember, academic study will always require independent work; attending lectures will never be enough to be successful on your programme, and these activities will help to deepen your knowledge and understanding of the issues under scrutiny and give you practice at working on your own.

You might want to think about completing these activities as part of your personal development plan (PDP) or portfolio. After completing the activity, write it up in your PDP or portfolio in a section devoted to that particular skill, then look back over time to see how far you are developing. You can also do more of the activities for a key skill that you have identified a weakness in, which will help build your skill and confidence in this area.

We hope you find this book useful, and that it challenges you to critically think about medicines use in modern healthcare.

Paul, Ben and Simon

Chapter 1   Finding reliable information about medicines

NMC Future Nurse: Standards of Proficiency for Registered Nurses

This chapter will address the following platforms and proficiencies:

Platform 1: Being an accountable professional

At the point of registration, the registered nurse will be able to:

1.8   demonstrate the knowledge, skills and ability to think critically when applying evidence and drawing on experience to make evidence informed decisions in all situations.
1.15   demonstrate the numeracy, literacy, digital and technological skills required to meet the needs of people in their care to ensure safe and effective nursing practice.
1.20   safely demonstrate evidence-based practice in all skills and procedures stated in Annexes A and B.

Chapter aims

By the end of this chapter you should be able to:

1.   Better understand the layout of the British National Formulary (BNF) and Summary of Product Characteristics (SmPC), and the information that they contain.
2.   Better understand the terminology used in the BNF and SmPC.
3.   Use the BNF and SmPC to obtain information about medicines.

Introduction

Medicines are one of the most commonly used interventions in healthcare, and their effective use and management can be associated with significant patient benefit. However, medicines use is not without risk, and ensuring the safe and effective use of medicines requires knowledge and understanding of many different aspects related to both your patient and their medicines. Some of this knowledge will be acquired through familiarity with the use of medicines in practice. However, given the broad range and increasingly complex nature of many medicines, it is not possible to have a complete understanding of every medicine. It is therefore important to know where to obtain reliable information about medicines and their use, when you encounter a patient who is prescribed a medicine that is unfamiliar to you.

This chapter introduces you to two fundamental sources of medicines information that are available in the United Kingdom, the British National Formulary (BNF) (and British National Formulary for Children [BNFC]), and the Summary of Product Characteristics (SmPC or SPC). These resources will be used in many of the activities throughout this book.

The British National Formulary (BNF) and British National Formulary for Children (BNFC)

The BNF (and BNFC) provides healthcare professionals with reliable, up-to-date, practice-oriented information about the use of medicines. It includes guidance on many aspects of medicines management including administration, dispensing and prescribing, as well as information on individual medicines. The information is drawn from several sources including manufacturers' product literature, the broader medical and pharmaceutical literature, and information and guidance from UK health departments, regulators and professional bodies.

Navigating the BNF

Activity 1.1   Research

The BNF and BNFC can be accessed in paper format, but they are also available via the internet and via an app for Android and Apple users. Try to find a paper copy of the BNF, and also download the app for your smartphone or tablet, or go to the BNF website (https://bnf.nice.org.uk) if you have access to a computer.

Compare how the information in the BNF is presented in the paper and electronic format. What are the different sections in the paper version, and is the layout the same in the electronic version?

As this activity is based on your own research, no outline answer is provided at the end of the chapter, however the text below highlights some key points.

The paper version of the BNF could be considered as having three sections that are particularly important when managing medicines. At the front of the book, there is advice about prescribing, and the use of medicines in patients with different characteristics (e.g. medicine use and renal function, medicines and palliative care). Next are chapters detailing medicines used in treating different body systems, such as respiratory, cardiovascular and central nervous system. Finally, there are the appendices. We'll be using Appendix 1, relating to drug interactions, later in this book.

The same information is available in the electronic versions, although at first glance, it is presented slightly differently. You can find specific information using the search function. However, the information corresponding to the start of the paper BNF is included under 'Medicines Guidance', the information in the chapters on body systems can be found under 'Drugs' and 'Treatment summaries', and the information in Appendix 1 under 'Interactions'. We'll explore these sections in a little more detail below.

All versions have a section describing how the content is arranged, which provides a useful guide to using the BNF, and explains how it is constructed.

Medicines guidance in the BNF

Activity 1.2   Evidence-based practice

Use the Medicines Guidance sections indicated [in brackets] to answer the following questions:

1. [Guidance on intravenous infusions] How many drugs should usually be added to an infusion container?
2. [Antimicrobial stewardship] What is antimicrobial resistance, and what contributes to its development?
3. [Adverse reactions to drugs] In what proportion of patients does a 'very common' side effect occur?
4. [Prescribing in pregnancy] Between which weeks of pregnancy is the greatest risk of drug induced congenital malformations?
5. [Prescribing in children] Why is the risk of drug toxicity increased in neonates?
6. [Prescribing in renal impairment] How can many of the problems associated with using drugs in patients with reduced kidney function be avoided?

An outline answer is given at the end of this chapter.

The Medicines Guidance sections usually give general advice or an overview of the issues encountered when managing medicines for particular patient groups (such as pregnancy in the activity above) or in particular situations. In the paper version of the

BNF, the Medicine Guidance sections can be found at the front of the book, whilst they are found under 'Guidance' or 'Medicines Guidance' in the app and online versions respectively. Similar content is available in the BNFC. More specific information relating to individual drugs can be found later in the BNF.

Drug monographs and treatment summaries in the BNF

Activity 1.3   Evidence-based practice

Search for the antidepressant drug sertraline in a paper or electronic version of the BNF, and then answer the following questions:

1. What do you think is meant by the term 'indication', and what are the indications for sertraline?
2. What is the initial dose of sertraline, for an adult patient, for the treatment of depressive illness?
3. Which of the following is a common or very common side effect of sertraline?

    a. Coma
    b. Gastrointestinal disorders
    c. Hiccups
    d. Diabetes mellitus

4. What do you think is meant by the term 'contra-indication', and which of the following is a contra-indication to sertraline use?

    a. Eczema
    b. High blood pressure (hypertension)
    c. Overactive thyroid (hyperthyroidism)
    d. Poorly controlled epilepsy

5. Can sertraline be used in patients with severe hepatic impairment?
6. What medicinal forms of sertraline are available?

An outline answer is given at the end of this chapter.

When you search for a specific drug in the BNF, you will usually be directed to the 'Drug monograph' for that particular drug. In the example in Activity 1.3, you should have found the monograph for sertraline. The drug monographs are organised in chapters according to body systems and contain information specific to the use of an individual drug.

The information contained in the monograph varies slightly from drug to drug, but will include what condition(s) it is used to treat (the indication), situations where it should not be used (contra-indications), situations where it needs to be used with care (cautions), as well as information about its side effects, including any important safety warnings that might have been issued. Where relevant, guidance on use of the drug in patients who have impaired hepatic (liver) or renal (kidney) function is included, along with information for its use in patients who are pregnant or breast feeding. At the end of the monograph, you will find a list of the available medicinal forms of the drug (such as tablets or injections), along with their legal classification (see Chapter 3 for more detail).

If you are administering a medicine to a patient, the information contained in the monograph can help you to ensure that you are giving the correct dose, and that there are no reasons to avoid that particular drug for your patient. See Chapter 4 for further information relating to medicine formulation, routes of administration and dosage.

Activity 1.4   Evidence-based practice

Search for the 'Antidepressant drug' treatment summary in an electronic version of the BNF, or the section on 'depression' in a paper copy of the BNF, and then answer the following questions:

1. What are the major classes of antidepressant drug?
2. Which group of antidepressants has better efficacy?
3. Which group of antidepressants is better tolerated, and is usually used first line for the treatment of depression?
4. For how long should antidepressant treatment be continued after a patient has achieved remission?
5. What symptoms might suggest that a patient has antidepressant induced hyponatraemia?

An outline answer is given at the end of this chapter.

As well as finding drug monographs in the body systems chapters of the paper version of the BNF and BNFC, you will also find 'Treatment summaries'. Whilst the drug monograph contains information about a specific drug, the 'Treatment summaries' contain information about a group of drugs, or the management of a certain condition. It is important to use both the monograph, and any relevant treatment summaries to inform decisions about medicines management, as the information contained in each will not necessarily be duplicated. For example, contra-indications or side effects that apply to a whole class of drug might be found in the treatment summary, rather than the individual monograph.

In the paper version of the BNF, the treatment summary is usually found before relevant drug monographs. In Activity 1.4, the treatment summary for depression precedes the monographs for the individual antidepressant drugs. In the online BNF, the treatment summaries can be accessed from the home page, and are also listed next to relevant drug monographs, whilst in the app they can be accessed directly.

Drug interactions in the BNF

Activity 1.5   Evidence-based practice

Access the 'Interactions' using an electronic version of the BNF, or Appendix 1 (Interactions) in a paper copy of the BNF, and then answer the following question:

Which of the following has a severe interaction with sertraline?

a.   Atenolol
b.   Ibuprofen
c.   Paracetamol
d.   Warfarin

As this activity is based on your own observations, no outline answer is provided at the end of this chapter, however the text below explains how to find the answer to this question.

When using an electronic version (app or online) version of the BNF, searching for interactions is relatively straightforward. You can search for the drug that you are interested in (e.g. sertraline), and an alphabetical list of interacting drugs is provided. There may also be a colour code or text stating whether the interaction can be considered mild, moderate, severe or of unknown severity. From the list in Activity 1.5, neither atenolol nor paracetamol are listed as interacting with sertraline, ibuprofen has an interaction, but it is not categorised as severe, whereas warfarin has an interaction with sertraline, which is categorised as severe.

Searching Appendix 1 in the paper BNF can be more complicated. Drugs are listed alphabetically, but they are also grouped. When you look for sertraline, you are directed to SSRIs (the group of antidepressants to which sertraline belongs). You can then look through the alphabetical list of drugs that interact with SSRIs. However, this is only part of the process. At the start of the entry for SSRIs, you are also referred to certain 'Tables'. These can be found at the start of Appendix 1 and contain further lists of drugs that can interact with your drug of interest. Sertraline has antiplatelet effects and can therefore interact with ibuprofen. Furthermore, the BNF notes that drugs with antiplatelet effects can also interact with drugs with anticoagulant effects such as warfarin. Interactions with ibuprofen and warfarin are therefore identified; however, no indication of the severity of these interactions is given.

The Summary of Product Characteristics (SmPC or SPC)

The drug development process generates large amounts of data about a medicine, which are submitted as evidence to the Medicines and Healthcare products Regulatory Agency

(MHRA) when the manufacturer applies to sell the medicine in the UK. A summary of this data, which is useful to healthcare professionals, can be found in a document called the Summary of Product Characteristics (referred to as the SmPC or sometimes SPC). The SmPC is a useful resource, containing detailed information about the licensed use of the relevant drug. SmPCs can be accessed via the Electronic Medicines Compendium website (www.medicines.org.uk/emc), where you can also find Patient Information Leaflets (PILs). These contain information that is specifically aimed at patients.

The SmPC is divided into ten sections. The first three parts describe the name, active ingredient and presentation of the medicine. The fifth part provides some information about the drug's pharmacology (how the drug works). This section can vary in the amount of information provided, with some SmPCs being very detailed, whereas others are less so. The sixth part lists the ingredients of the medicine, which can be useful if a patient has an allergy to a particular component. The final three parts provide regulatory details.

The fourth part of the SmPC provides information relating to the clinical use of the medicine. It will state the indications for the product (i.e. for what illness or condition the medicine can be used), age ranges of patients to which it can be given, how much should be given and at what time interval. It will list contra-indications and cautions, adverse effects, interactions with other drugs, and use of the drug in specific groups (such as during pregnancy). The information contained in this section is similar to that found in the BNF. However, it typically has more detail, with a brief explanation of the evidence that underpins these aspects.

Activity 1.6   Critical thinking

Go to the Electronic Medicines Compendium website and type 'Ramipril' into the search bar. Select the SmPC for one of the ramipril products and have a look at the information that it contains. An example can also be found at: www.medicines.org.uk/emc/product/8448/smpc

Compare this with the information provided in a PIL for ramipril, which can also be selected after accessing ramipril from the search bar. How are they different, and why might that be?

An outline answer is given at the end of the chapter.

Chapter summary

This chapter has focused on two fundamental sources of medicines information available in the UK (the BNF and SmPCs). Although a significant amount of information is available in these sources, decisions about medicines use also require clinical judgement. If you are unsure how to manage a patient's medicine, you should seek advice from a more experienced colleague, prescriber or pharmacist.

The format of the paper version of the BNF has changed over time. This chapter has been written making use of BNF 80, published in 2020. However, if you are using later versions, the layout may have changed, and the information been presented in a slightly different way. Similarly, the electronic versions may evolve over time. The evidence base supporting medicines use develops quickly, and it is important that you use the most up to date version of any reference source, to ensure that your decisions are made using current evidence.

Whilst the BNF and SmPCs are very useful, they are not the only sources of information regarding medicines and disease management. For example, the Clinical Knowledge Summaries website (https://cks.nice.org.uk) also provided by the UK's National Institute for Health and Care Excellence (NICE), provides information on common illnesses along with their relevant treatment pathways. An awareness of how to access reliable information and how to apply it effectively is key to safe medicines management. The resources identified should form the building blocks for further reading and ongoing professional development.

Activities: Brief outline answers

Activity 1.2 Evidence-based practice (page 6)

1. Only one drug should normally be added to an intravenous infusion fluid container. This information can be found under the 'Guideline' subheading in the 'Guidance on intravenous infusions', Medicines Guidance. However, it is important to note that you may encounter certain circumstances in practice, where medicines are combined prior to administration.

2. Antimicrobial resistance means that a drug used to treat infections caused by micro-organisms becomes less effective. Inappropriate use of antimicrobial drugs contributes to the development of antimicrobial resistance. This information can be found in the 'Overview' of the 'Antimicrobial stewardship', Medicines Guidance.

3. A 'very common' side effect occurs in more than one in ten patients treated with the drug. This information can be found in the 'Description of the frequency of side-effects' section of the 'Adverse reactions to drugs', Medicines Guidance.

4. The greatest risk of drug induced congenital malformations occurs between weeks three and eleven of pregnancy. This information can be found in the 'Overview' of the 'Prescribing in pregnancy', Medicines Guidance.

5. Reduced drug clearance and target organ sensitivity increase the risk of drug toxicity in neonates. This information can be found in the 'Overview' of the 'Prescribing in children', Medicines Guidance.

6. Reducing the dose or switching to an alternative drug can reduce the risk of problems associated with using drugs in patients with reduced kidney function. This information can be found in the 'Issues encountered in renal impairment' of the 'Prescribing in renal impairment', Medicines Guidance.

Activity 1.3 Evidence-based practice (page 7)

1. An indication is the reason a drug is used. At the time of writing, sertraline was indicated for the management of depressive illness, obsessive compulsive disorder, panic disorder, post-traumatic stress disorder and social anxiety disorder.

2. The initial dose for an adult for the treatment of depressive illness is 50mg.

3. Gastrointestinal disorders are a common or very common side effect of sertraline.

4. A contra-indication is a condition or situation where a medicine should not be used. Poorly controlled epilepsy is a contra-indication to sertraline use.

5. Sertraline should be avoided in patients with severe hepatic impairment.

6. Sertraline is available as a tablet, although special order manufacturers can supply oral suspensions. Special order manufacturers will make small batches of medicines that are not typically made by the original manufacturer. In the example above, a special order manufacturer will make sertraline oral suspension whereas the original manufacturer only makes tablets. These medicines are often called 'specials' and are typically a lot more expensive to purchase than the standard medicine.

Activity 1.4 Evidence-based practice (page 8)

1. The major classes of antidepressant drug are the tricyclic and related antidepressants, the selective serotonin re-uptake inhibitors (SSRIs), and the monoamine oxidase inhibitors (MAOIs). This classification is based upon the chemistry of the drugs (tricyclic), or their mechanism of action (SSRIs and MAOIs). However, there are a number of different types of antidepressant, and dividing them into only three broad categories does not capture the diversity of this group of drugs.

2. There is little evidence that any group of antidepressants has better efficacy than another.

3. Selective serotonin re-uptake inhibitors (SSRIs) are better tolerated, and usually used first line for the treatment of depression.

4. Antidepressant treatment should usually be continued for at least six months after a patient has achieved remission.

5. Developing drowsiness, confusion or convulsions might suggest that a patient has antidepressant induced hyponatraemia.

Activity 1.6 Critical thinking (page 10)

The patient information leaflet (PIL) and Summary of product characteristics (SmPC) are intended to be read by patients and healthcare professionals respectively. Much of the information presented in each document is similar, such as what the medication is used for (indication), when not to take it, contraindications, warnings (cautions), interactions with other medicines, doses and side effects. However, the way in which the information is presented is slightly different, and the SmPC contains a section on the pharmacology of the drug, and some details from clinical studies. SmPCs vary in the amount of pharmacological and study data that they include, but they will typically describe the drug's mechanism of action, and state how it is absorbed and eliminated from the body.

Further reading

The British National Formulary. Available at https://bnf.nice.org.uk

A standard reference source for all aspects of medicines management.

Clinical Knowledge Summaries. Available at https://cks.nice.org.uk

Information relating to the management of common conditions encountered in primary care.

Chapter 2   What is a medicine?

Chapter aims

By the end of this chapter you should be able to:

1. Explain the difference between a medicinal product and a drug.
2. Identify medicinal products that patients are taking.
3. List and utilise some resources used to classify and manage medicines.

(Continued)

(Continued)

4. Describe different mechanisms of drug action.
5. Describe the development process of a medicine.
6. Apply knowledge of the principles of safety, quality and efficacy when giving advice to a service user/patient.

Introduction

This chapter will begin with a case study containing an extract from Barrie's medicine administration chart, which shows some of the different types of treatment that your patients may be taking. The first part of the chapter explains how medicines are defined and explores how you can obtain reliable information about medicines. Later in the chapter, you will start to explore some of the ways in which drugs work (their pharmacology), and how they are developed for human use, to maximise safety, quality and efficacy (to ensure the drug works as it is designed to do). You will also reflect upon the ways in which patients choose to access medicines, and some of the problems that might be associated with this.

Case study

Barrie's medicines

Medicines to be given regularly				Dose		
1	Date 27/5/22	Drug and form Ramipril capsule	Route Oral			breakfast
						lunch
	Prescriber's signature Dr RSY	Other directions				teatime
					10mg	night
2	Date 27/5/22	Drug and form Amlodipine tablet	Route Oral			breakfast
						lunch
	Prescriber's signature Dr RSY	Other directions				teatime
					5mg	night
3	Date 27/5/22	Drug and form St John's Wort capsule (284mg)	Route Oral	One		breakfast
						lunch
	Prescriber's signature Dr RSY	Other directions Patient's own				teatime
						night
4	Date 27/5/22	Drug and form Centrum for Men capsule	Route Oral	One		breakfast
						lunch
	Prescriber's signature Dr RSY	Other directions Patient's own				teatime
						night

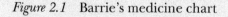

Figure 2.1   Barrie's medicine chart

Barrie is a 56-year-old man with high blood pressure (hypertension) and has come into hospital because over the last few months his blood pressure has been difficult to control. Although he doesn't have any particular symptoms, his GP has been concerned and has referred him to the cardiology consultant. Figure 2.1 shows a list of medicines taken by Barrie. The form used to list the medicines is similar to the medicine administration charts used in hospital in the UK. The list of medicines taken by Barrie includes two licensed medicinal products for his blood pressure (ramipril and amlodipine). He also takes two products that he has bought from a health food store: a herbal product to help his mood (St John's Wort), and a vitamin and mineral supplement (Centrum Men®).

Medicinal products (medicines)

Medicines can broadly be defined as products that are used to prevent or treat disease in humans, or which restore or modify a physiological process through a pharmacological or immunological action. A medicinal product may also be a substance used to diagnose a disease. In the UK, the legal definition of a medicinal product is found in the Human Medicines Regulations (2012). This is a piece of legislation that you can find on the government's website (www.legislation.gov.uk/uksi/2012/1916/contents/made).

Which of the products that Barrie is taking are medicinal products (medicines)?

In the list above, ramipril and amlodipine are medicinal products. They are intended to treat a disease (hypertension) and modify a physiological function through a pharmacological effect. In order to market and sell a medicinal product in the UK, a manufacturer must obtain a marketing authorisation (MA). The MA was previously known as a product licence, and you may still hear medicines referred to as 'licensed medicines'. To obtain an MA, medicines have to be manufactured, marketed and monitored to a regulatory standard. In the UK, MAs are granted by a government organisation called the Medicines and Healthcare products Regulatory Agency (MHRA). Before they can be granted an MA to market and sell a medicine, a manufacturer must carry out specific, scientific testing procedures to show that their product meets the required standard. This is a rigorous process that centres on demonstrating that the product can be manufactured to the required thresholds of safety, quality and efficacy. Further information on the drug development process can be found later in this chapter.

Healthcare professionals can have confidence that a licensed medicine will have the clinical benefit that is intended, because of the evidence presented to obtain an MA. Licensed medicines are used to treat major disease and a range of acute and chronic conditions.

In demonstrating efficacy, the manufacturer presents evidence that the medicine will have the clinical action required, e.g. a medicine which lowers blood pressure will actually lower blood pressure. They must additionally provide evidence that the product has an appropriate safety profile, i.e. the potential risks do not outweigh the benefits, and they must be able to demonstrate that they can produce the medicine to good standards of quality with consistent processes applied. The process of producing a medicine to these standards requires significant investment and scientific rigour to ensure safety, quality and efficacy.

Whilst marketing authorisation helps to reassure healthcare professionals about the quality, efficacy and safety of a product, it is not always possible to use a licensed product for a particular condition. This might be because a company hasn't applied for marketing authorisation in the country where the product is being used. In this circumstance, a product from a different country that meets the need of the patient could be given. This would be an example of the use of an 'unlicensed medicine'. Although not illegal, the implications for healthcare professionals when using such products are different to when using a licensed medicine. In particular, there should be no available licensed alternative that meets the patient's needs, there should be sufficient evidence to support the use of the unlicensed medicine, and patients should have enough information to make an informed choice regarding the treatment.

In certain fields of medicine (for example paediatrics and mental health), it is relatively common to encounter the 'off-label' use of medicines. In contrast to 'unlicensed' usage discussed above, 'off-label' refers to the use of a medicine outside of the terms of the MA. This might include the use of the medicine at a dose that is outside the normal range, or for an indication not included in the MA. As MA will be in place for a medicine being used off label, healthcare professionals can be reassured about the quality of the medicine. However, other considerations will be the same as those for unlicensed medicines noted above. Off-label and unlicensed medicines have been associated with an increased risk of adverse effects, and additional care is needed in these aspects of medicines use.

Herbal remedies

Herbal remedies such as Barrie's St John's Wort are not classed as medicinal products but are nevertheless subject to controls by the MHRA. The MHRA hold a list of herbal remedies that hold a Traditional Herbal Registration (THR). Before a herbal remedy can be marketed in the UK it must be listed on the THR. THR is only granted if the product is sold to treat minor health conditions where medical supervision is not required. If a traditional herbal medicine claims to treat major or serious health conditions, the manufacturer is required to apply for a Marketing Authorisation (as with a medicinal product). Figure 2.2 illustrates how a herbal product is being used to treat a minor condition (low mood) rather than major depression.

What is contained in this product and for what conditions should it be used?
This herbal product contains an extract of St John's Wort (a natural herb). This is a traditional herbal remedy that is used to alleviate symptoms of a mild low mood and mild anxiety. The evidence for its use is based on traditional use.
Caution, before you take this product
Do not take this product if you are *Under 18 years of age, *About to have a surgical procedure *Have allergies to any of the ingredients, *If you are trying to get pregnant, are pregnant or breast feeding, *Receiving phototherapy treatment or if your skin is sensitive to sunlight (photosensitivity) *suffering from depression If a Medical expert such as a doctor or psychiatrist has informed you that you are suffering from or have a diagnosis of depression – please do not use this product If you think you are depressed – Please talk to a doctor before taking this product

Figure 2.2   Two extracts from the Patient Information Leaflet (PIL) for St John's Wort

There are some ingredients found in herbal products that are banned or restricted from manufacture or sale in the UK. These ingredients have evidence that they are toxic (and are therefore not safe), examples include *Atropa belladonna* and *Akebia quintata (Mutong)*. Some herbal remedies (e.g. St John's Wort) can affect the way in which other medicines work. Just because something is a plant-based remedy, doesn't mean that it is necessarily safe or that it can be used without consideration of a person's other medicines. This is particularly important to consider, as patients can buy these remedies themselves without medical supervision, and you may not always be aware that they are taking them.

Food supplements

The vitamin product (Centrum Men®), taken by Barrie, is a Food Supplement, not a medicine. Food supplements are defined by EU law as:

> *foodstuffs the purpose of which is to supplement the normal diet, and which are concentrated sources of nutrients or other substances with a nutritional or physiological effect, alone or in combination, marketed in dose form.*

> Further information is available at: www.gov.uk/government/
> publications/food-supplements-guidance-and-faqs

Food supplements are not regulated in the same way as medicines and cannot make any claim to prevent or cure a specific disease or illness. In the UK, each of the devolved nations has responsibility for administering regulations relating to these products.

Although Barrie's vitamin preparation is not an example of a medicine by legal definition, it does illustrate one of the broader approaches used to treat human disease. Many medicinal products that you will encounter in practice will replace an absent or depleted substance in the body. To illustrate this point, consider type 1 diabetes, where the pancreas is not capable of producing the hormone insulin. Without insulin from an external source the Type I diabetic patient would not be able to survive. Treatment uses injections of manufactured insulin, which has a similar action to the body's own insulin but a slightly different chemical structure.

There are many examples of medicines that are found in clinical practice that are essentially replacement therapies, for example, hormone replacement therapies, treatments for hypothyroidism such as levothyroxine, and colecalciferol (vitamin D). In this case, the vitamin D has a therapeutic effect and is treating medical deficiency and must therefore have marketing authorisation. This is in contrast to the Centrum Men®, which is used for supplementation alone. Some other examples of medicines and their actions are shown in Table 2.1, and these are explored in the section 'How drugs work' later in this chapter.

The difference between medicinal products and drugs

So far in this chapter, we have been talking about medicines. However, when working in practice, you will hear people talking about 'drugs', 'drug rounds' and 'drug charts', and the terms medicine and drug are often used interchangeably. The following section will explain the difference between a medicine and a drug, beginning with a case study.

Case study

Sonia, a 34-year-old woman, comes to the surgery to see the practice nurse for a review of her oral contraceptive. Her box of tablets is below.

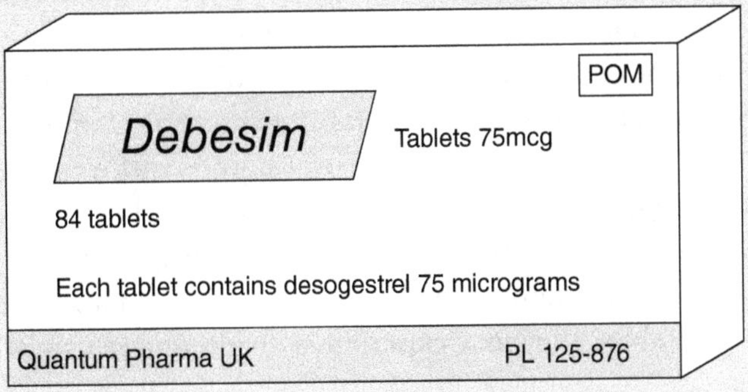

Figure 2.3 Sonia's tablet box

Activity 2.1 Evidence-based practice and research

Looking at the box of tablets in the case study above, use the BNF online (available at https://bnf.nice.org.uk) to find:

1. What desogestrel is used for?
2. What medicinal forms of desogestrel are available?
3. What dose is used?

An outline answer is given at the end of this chapter.

What is the significance of 'Tablets' and '75mcg' written on Sonia's Debesim medicine container?

A 'medicine' or 'medicinal product' is the form in which a drug is given to a patient. Medicines can take a number of different forms, including those intended to be taken by mouth such as tablets, capsules and liquids, and those intended to be given by other routes such as suppositories, creams and injections. As you may have found whilst completing Activity 2.2, the form (also called a formulation) of Sonia's medicine is a tablet; this is specified on the container.

The medicine formulation consists of a specific amount of the drug, as well as a number of other ingredients. The drug is the active ingredient and is responsible for the therapeutic effect. The amount of drug in the medicine is important, as the patient must take a specific amount (or dose) each day. The amount of drug is commonly expressed as a unit of weight, such as grams (g), milligrams (mg), or micrograms (mcg). Sonia's medicine contains 75mcg of the drug desogestrel. The dose will often depend upon what the drug is being used to treat. In the case of desogestrel, there is only one dose in the BNF.

The other ingredients in the medicine will depend on the formulation type. For medicines taken orally, these may include colourings, flavourings and preservatives. These other ingredients do not contribute to the therapeutic effect, but help to enable the drug to be given to the patient in an acceptable form. For example, flavourings may help to mask the taste of the drug and make oral liquids more palatable for children. Although these other ingredients do not contribute to the therapeutic effect, they can sometimes be responsible for unpleasant or adverse reactions to the medicine. For example, some tablets may contain colourings, to which some patients might be allergic. If the patient takes the tablet, they may experience an allergic reaction.

Medicine names

Medicines are typically known by more than one name; usually a generic name, and a brand name.

The generic name is also known as the international non-proprietary name (INN), and sometimes in the UK, the British Approved Name (BAN). It is the name of the active ingredient responsible for the therapeutic effect (the drug). In most cases the INN and BAN are the same and the INN is used to identify the drug. However, an important exception is 'epinephrine' (the INN), which is known in the UK as 'adrenaline' (the BAN).

The INN is a globally recognised name and facilitates identification of the drug by healthcare professionals. In the example above, 'desogestrel' is the generic name (and INN) of the drug, and you should have been able to find it in the BNF. A generic medicine contains the same active ingredient as the branded product, but because the costs associated with producing it are much lower, generic medicines are usually cheaper than the branded original.

The brand name is a name invented by the manufacturer (in the case above 'Debesim') and is used when marketing the medicine. You should have been able to find different brand names of desogestrel under medicinal forms in the BNF, including Cerazette® and Cerelle®. When a manufacturer is developing a medicine (see 'How vaccines and other medicines are developed' below for further information on the drug development process), they apply for a patent. The patent prevents other companies from selling the same medicine for a certain period of time. During this time, the medicine will typically only be available as the brand-named product. Once the manufacturer's patent for the medicine has expired, another company can market the drug, but not using the original brand name. In this case, the generic name will typically be used (hence the term 'Generic Medicine'). Eventually, the brand-named medicine may stop being made, as cheaper alternatives take over.

How drugs work

Now that we have discussed how medicines are defined and named, we can start to think about how drugs work. We have already seen that some drugs replace substances that our bodies are lacking. However, many drugs can modify physiological processes in the body. These are outlined below, beginning with a case study.

Case study

Harry's medicines

Harry has hypertension, which means that his blood pressure is higher than it should be. This can cause damage to his organs and could result in serious health consequences if not adequately controlled. The medicines Harry is taking to control his blood pressure are shown below.

Name:	Harry Browne		DOB: 5/6/1958
Condition(s):	High blood pressure		
Medicine	Formulation/route	Dose	Frequency
Atenolol	Tablet	25mg	Once a day
Ramipril	Capsule	2.5mg	Once a day

Figure 2.4 Harry's medicines

To manage his hypertension Harry is taking two drugs that lower his blood pressure, atenolol and ramipril. Both atenolol and ramipril can be classified as anti-hypertensive drugs, however whilst this describes the effect of the drug (reducing hypertension) it does not consider the way in which they achieve this effect (their mechanisms of action).

Mechanism of action

As described in the section at the beginning of the chapter 'How are medicines defined?', part of the definition of a medicinal product relates to '*restoring, correcting or modifying a physiological function by exerting a pharmacological, immunological or metabolic action*'. In order to manage drugs effectively it is important to understand how they work. This is often described as the drug's 'mechanism of action' or more technically its 'pharmacodynamics'. There are a number of different ways in which a drug can exert its action, but for many drugs this involves hijacking or disrupting existing control mechanisms within the body.

Drugs acting on receptors

As an example of a mechanism of action, look back at the case study and the Atenolol tablets on his medication list. How does Atenolol work? Atenolol is part of a group of drugs called beta-blockers. Like many drugs, beta-blockers work by disrupting the body's normal control systems, in this instance, the sympathetic nervous system. As part of the normal control of blood pressure the sympathetic nervous system releases the chemical noradrenaline, which stimulates the heart. This increases heart rate and contractility, raising blood pressure. The noradrenaline stimulates the heart by binding to specialised proteins called receptors (in this case adrenoceptors) embedded in the cell membrane of the cardiac cells. When these receptors are bound to, they activate cellular mechanisms within the cell, resulting in increased heart rate. Beta-blockers are also able to bind to the adrenoceptor, but when bound, do not activate the cellular mechanisms. Furthermore, whilst the beta-blocker is bound to the receptor the noradrenaline cannot bind and therefore cannot affect the heart. As a result, blood pressure is reduced.

Unlike beta-blockers, which prevent activation of the receptor by noradrenaline, some drugs that bind to receptors produce a response in the associated cellular mechanism, just like the body's own chemicals. These are called agonists, whilst chemicals that bind to receptors and cause no effect are called antagonists. Agonists and antagonists of different receptors are used throughout healthcare. Agonist drugs are used to stimulate a process in the body (for example salbutamol, which causes bronchodilation and is used in the treatment of asthma), whilst antagonists are used to block a process (such as antihistamines, which block histamine receptors and prevent allergic responses).

The body uses a multitude of different signalling molecules throughout the body (i.e. neurotransmitters and hormones). These signalling molecules are only able to bind to their own specific type of receptor, which is why hormones might only affect one part of the body even though they are dispersed throughout the whole body.

In some instances, the body might have different types of receptor for the same agonist. For example, noradrenaline causes peripheral arterioles to constrict by stimulating one type of receptor, called the alpha-adrenergic receptor, whilst on the heart, it stimulates a different type of receptor called the beta-adrenergic receptor. The different subtypes of receptor can be targeted, allowing us to use drugs that will only affect one type of receptor, reducing unwanted side effects. Beta-blockers, as the name suggests, selectively antagonise beta-adrenergic receptors rather than alpha-adrenergic receptors.

Drugs acting on enzymes

Harry's ramipril is part of a group of drugs called ACE inhibitors, which disrupt the action of the renin-angiotensin-aldosterone-system (RAAS). Specifically, it inhibits an enzyme called Angiotensin Converting Enzyme or ACE. This enzyme converts a substance called angiotensin I, which does nothing, into angiotensin II, which has powerful blood-pressure-raising properties. If the action of ACE is inhibited, angiotensin II will not be produced, and the blood pressure will not rise.

Enzymes represent another very important target for drugs to act upon. Enzymes are biological catalysts that facilitate most of the chemical reactions that happen in the body. These enzymes are responsible for making things and breaking things; for example, manufacturing substances within the body (such as Angiotensin II) or breaking substances down. As different enzymes are used to catalyse different chemical reactions it is possible to produce drugs that target one type of enzyme and thereby inhibit one specific reaction.

If an enzyme is responsible for producing a substance, inhibiting that enzyme will prevent that substance from being created and thereby prevent any action or effect that that substance has (such as the ACE inhibitor preventing the production of angiotensin II discussed above). If an enzyme is responsible for breaking something down, inhibiting that enzyme will prevent the substance from being broken down and keep it around in the body for longer. An example of this is Dipeptidyl peptidase-4 (DPP-4) inhibitors, which inhibit the enzyme responsible for breaking down Glucagon like peptide-1 (GLP-1). GLP-1 is responsible for stimulating the pancreas to produce insulin. Inhibiting the DPP-4 enzyme results in raised levels of GLP-1, which results in more insulin being released from the pancreas, which is very useful in the treatment of type 2 diabetes.

Activity 2.2   Evidence-based practice and research

Look up the following drugs in the BNF and try to identify their mechanisms of action.

1. Losartan
2. Vardenafil
3. Allopurinol
4. Montelukast

An outline answer is given at the end of this chapter.

Case study

Sally's medicines

Sally has depression and anxiety and is taking two medicines (diazepam and escitalopram) to help her manage her condition.

(Continued)

(Continued)

Name:	Sally Wilkinson		DOB: 23/9/1977
Condition(s):	Depression and anxiety		
Medicine	Formulation/route	Dose	Frequency
Diazepam	Tablet	5mg	Once a day at night
Escitalopram	Tablet	2.5mg	Once a day

Figure 2.5 Sally's medicines

The medicines that Sally is taking are intended to either increase nerve cell (neuronal) excitation (relieving some of the symptoms of depression) or reduce neuronal excitation (relieving some of the symptoms of anxiety). Whilst these two actions seem contradictory, they are affecting different neurotransmitters in different pathways of the brain.

Both escitalopram and diazepam work by enhancing the action of neurotransmitters in the brain. Escitalopram enhances the action of the neurotransmitter serotonin and diazepam enhances the action of the neurotransmitter GABA (gamma aminobutyric acid) with the intention of returning their respective levels of activity to normal.

Drugs acting on Transport Proteins

Like many drugs acting on the central nervous system, escitalopram affects the way in which nerve cells (neurones) send signals or messages to each other. A neurone can receive, conduct and transmit signals to adjacent neurones by releasing neurotransmitters (endogenous agonists). Synaptic transmission takes place in a fraction of a second. When a neurone is activated, neurotransmitters are released from the terminal area of the presynaptic neurone and diffuse across the microscopic distances of the synaptic cleft. The neurotransmitter then binds to and stimulates receptors in the membrane of the post synaptic neurone. After they have stimulated the post synaptic neurone, the neurotransmitters are removed from the synaptic cleft, either through enzymatic degradation or by being 'pumped' by transport proteins out of the synaptic cleft and back into the presynaptic neurone.

Escitalopram is one of a group of drugs called selective serotonin reuptake inhibitors (SSRIs). It works by inhibiting the Serotonin Reuptake Transporter (SERT), which is normally responsible for the re-uptake of the neurotransmitter serotonin back into the presynaptic neurone. By blocking this transport protein, escitalopram prevents serotonin from being removed from the synaptic cleft, prolonging its action and raising the patient's mood.

Drugs acting on ion channels

Diazepam works by enhancing the brain's own 'braking mechanism' and enhancing the action of the inhibitory neurotransmitter GABA (gamma amino butyric acid).

The excitation of a neurone is a product of the movement of charged ions (e.g. Na^+, K^+ and Cl^-) into and out of the cell. This is only possible due to specialised transmembrane proteins, which form pores or channels to allow substances to pass from one side of the cell membrane to the other. A 'depolarisation' of cell is initiated by the binding of an excitatory neurotransmitter, which facilitates the opening of ion channels, resulting in an influx of positively charged ions (e.g. Na^+), which makes the interior of the cell more positively charged. GABAergic neurones work against this by releasing the inhibitory neurotransmitter GABA, which activates GABA-mediated chloride channels and allows an influx of negatively charged chloride (Cl^-) ions into the cell. This makes the interior of the cell more negative and less likely to be activated. Diazepam and other benzodiazepines enhance the action of GABA and therefore allow more chloride ions into the cell, reducing its activity.

Other drugs with similar mechanisms of action

Membrane-spanning proteins such as ion channels are an important target for a number of drugs. Cell membranes are intended to keep the inside and outside of the cell separate. Water soluble molecules such as sugars, ions, neurotransmitters and hormones can only cross the membrane with the help of these specialised transmembrane proteins. The proteins either actively transport the substance from one side to the other, or form channels that allow the substance to flow along the concentration gradient from one side of the membrane to the other. Blocking or inhibiting these transport proteins can have a tremendous impact upon the function of tissues and organs.

Other examples

Proton Pump Inhibitors (PPIs) such as lansoprazole or omeprazole inhibit the transport protein responsible for 'pumping' hydrogen ions (which are what make things acidic) out of parietal cells and into the stomach, creating stomach acid. By blocking these transporters, the contents of the stomach become less acidic and dyspepsia (indigestion) is reduced.

Digoxin, one of the most widely recognised antiarrhythmic drugs, acts upon the transporter that pumps sodium and potassium into and out of cardiac myocytes (muscle cells). By influencing the electrophysiology of cardiac tissue, this helps to maintain the normal rhythm of the heart.

Dapagliflozin, empagliflozin and canagliflozin are part of a group of drugs called SGLT-2 inhibitors. SGLT-2 stands for **S**odium-**g**lucose-**t**ransporter-2, which is a transporter found in the kidney, and is responsible for pumping glucose out of the urine, and back into the body. SGLT-2 inhibitors block this reuptake of glucose, causing it to be lost from the body in the urine. This can be an effective way of lowering blood sugar in diabetes.

Drug	Therapeutic Target	Action	Examples of Indications
Adrenaline (epinephrine)	Alpha and beta adrenergic receptors	Agonist	Cardiopulmonary resuscitation, acute hypotension
Morphine	Opioid mu receptor	Agonist	Pain
Prednisolone	Glucocorticoid receptor	Agonist	Acute exacerbation of asthma, suppression of inflammatory disorders, local joint inflammation, ulcerative colitis
Salbutamol	$Beta_2$ adrenergic receptor	Agonist	Acute bronchospasm, acute asthma
Bisoprolol	$Beta_1$ adrenergic receptor	Antagonist	Angina, hypertension, adjunct in heart failure
Cetirizine	Histamine H_1 receptor	Antagonist	Relief of allergy e.g. hayfever
Losartan	Angiotensin II AT_1 receptor	Antagonist	Heart failure, hypertension
Risperidone	Dopamine D_2 receptor/ serotonin $5\text{-}HT_{2A}$ receptor	Antagonist	Psychosis, schizophrenia
Tiotropium	Muscarinic acetylcholine receptor	Antagonist	Maintenance of chronic obstructive pulmonary disease
Aspirin	Cyclo-oxygenase enzyme	Inhibitor	Analgesia, anti-inflammatory, prevention of cardiovascular events
Atorvastatin	HMG CoA reductase enzyme	Inhibitor	Primary hypercholesterolaemia, prevention of cardiovascular events
Donepezil	Acetylcholinesterase enzyme	Inhibitor	Dementia in Alzheimer's disease
Ramipril	Angiotensin converting enzyme	Inhibitor	Heart failure, hypertension
Rivaroxaban	Factor Xa enzyme	Inhibitor	Treatment of deep vein thrombosis, prevention of stroke in non-valvular atrial fibrillation
Sitagliptin	Dipeptidylpeptidase–4 (DPP–4) enzyme	Inhibitor	Type 2 diabetes
Diltiazem	Voltage-gated calcium channel	Blocker	Hypertension, angina prophylaxis
Lorazepam	$GABA_A$ ligand gated chloride channel	Positive allosteric modulator	Anxiety
Lidocaine	Voltage-gated sodium channel	Blocker	Local anaesthesia
Ondansetron	Serotonin $5\text{-}HT_3$ ligand gated ion channel	Antagonist	Nausea

Drug	Therapeutic Target	Action	Examples of Indications
Dapagliflozin	Sodium glucose co-transporter 2	Inhibitor	Type 2 diabetes
Furosemide	Chloride ion transporter	Inhibitor	Oedema
Omeprazole	H+/K+ – ATPase (proton pump)	Inhibitor	Benign gastric ulceration, gastro-oesophageal reflux disease
Sertraline	Serotonin reuptake transporter	Inhibitor	Depression, obsessive compulsive disorder
Colecalciferol	Vitamin D_3	Replace	Deficiency
Ferrous fumarate	Iron	Replace	Iron–deficiency anaemia
Levodopa	Dopamine	Replace	Parkinson's disease
Levothyroxine	Triiodothyronine	Replace	Hypothyroidism
Thiamine	Vitamin B_1	Replace	Deficiency

Table 2.1 Commonly used drugs, and their mechanisms of action

How patients access medicines

Case study

During her consultation with the nurse, Sonia mentions that she hasn't been sleeping well recently. When the practice nurse asks her whether she needs any advice regarding the management of her insomnia, she replies that she has bought some diazepam from the internet and is hoping that will help. Sonia shows the packet to the practice nurse, who sees that it seems to be from a different country. The nurse can see the word 'diazepam', the number '10', and there is another name 'Maxsleep', which the nurse doesn't recognise.

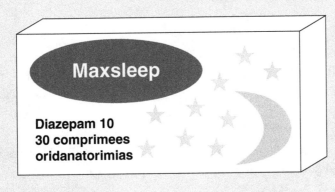

Maxsleep

Diazepam 10
30 comprimees
oridanatorimias

Figure 2.6 Sonia's Maxsleep tablets

As illustrated in the case study above, the ways in which people can obtain or access medicines is changing. As well as traditional routes such as visiting a community pharmacy (either to purchase over the counter medicines or to have a prescription dispensed), the internet has enabled access to medicines at the click of a button. Whilst this may be convenient and facilitates patient choice, it also presents certain challenges. You may need to advise your patients about these challenges. The following section outlines some things to consider.

If patients buy medicines from the internet, they may not be aware of the correct dose for their condition. Sonia's tablets contain 10mg of diazepam, which is equivalent to the highest strength of tablet available in the UK. However, unlike desogestrel, several different doses of diazepam can be used, depending upon the condition being treated. If Sonia takes too much diazepam, she may experience unpleasant (or adverse) effects. It is also possible that the medicine may not be suitable for Sonia due to other medical conditions that she may have. For medicines available in the UK, this information can be found under contra-indications and cautions in the BNF. Without seeking advice from a healthcare professional, Sonia might be unaware of this.

Sonia's box of oral contraceptive pills (Debesim) has been produced by a pharmaceutical company based in the UK. The quality of this medicine will have been assessed by the MHRA and granted a product licence. When buying medicines from the internet, it is possible that the brand supplied will not be one that is available in the UK. In the example above, the nurse was not familiar with the name Maxsleep, as it is not available in the UK. Furthermore, individuals may try to make money through selling counterfeit (fake) medicines. In these examples the medicine may not have been subject to the same testing as a UK licensed product. This could mean that the medicine may not have the correct active ingredient, the right amount of the active ingredient, or it may contain other toxic substances. This is a further risk of purchasing medicines from non-approved sources.

Other medicinal products
Vaccines

Case study

A patient named Mr Atkins received the following letter through the post.

Dear Mr Atkins,

Your annual flu vaccination is now due.

Flu vaccination provides the best protection against an unpredictable virus which infects many people and can cause serious illness and death each year.

Please phone the practice to book an appointment for your flu vaccination. The vaccination is free and recommended yearly for those most at risk from flu.

This includes:

- children aged 2 to 10 years old
- pregnant women

- anyone living with a long-term medical condition
- everyone aged 65 and over
- people with caring responsibilities

If there is someone you rely on to care for you, please ask them to contact their own GP Practice as they may be eligible for a free flu vaccination.

We look forward to seeing you soon.

Activity 2.3   Evidence-based practice and research

Look at the influenza vaccine 'Treatment summary' section of the BNF online and find out which medical conditions make people *at* high risk from influenza.

An outline answer is given at the end of this chapter.

Are vaccines medicines?

As you'll see in Chapter 7, vaccines are key to preventing many diseases. This is particularly important for vulnerable patients such as those with other illnesses, as you would have seen when completing Activity 2.5. The criteria used to classify medicinal products in the Human Medicines Regulations include a substance presented as having properties of preventing disease and a substance that modifies a physiological function by exerting an immunological action. Vaccines are designed to prevent disease by modifying an immune response and are therefore classified as medicinal products. Vaccines are developed and managed in a similar way to other medicines.

How vaccines and other medicines are developed

The development of most medicines is a long and expensive process. It has been estimated that the cost of bringing a new medicine to market between 2009 and 2014 was, on average, in excess of 900m US dollars (Wouters et al., 2020). Furthermore, for most medicines the process takes approximately 12 years (Mohsa and Greig, 2017). Once a potential drug molecule has been identified, it must be tested for safety, quality and efficacy before it can be granted approval (known as marketing authorisation or previously a licence) to be sold or marketed by the pharmaceutical company.

Once a chemical substance has been identified as a potential drug, it must first be tested in non-human models to assess its potential safety and efficacy. This is the pre-clinical development phase. The substance must also be formulated as a medicine that is suitable to be administered to humans. Due to the properties of the chemical substance, it may not be possible to formulate it as a medicine, and therefore it will not be suitable to develop further. If a drug shows evidence of safety and efficacy in preclinical studies, it will undergo testing in humans as an 'investigational medicinal product' (IMP) in four phases of clinical trials.

'Phase 1' clinical studies are designed to identify safety issues and characterise some of the pharmacological properties of the IMP. The initial 'First into human' studies will be done in a small number of healthy volunteers (typically younger males), or sometime patients, who will be given a single dose of the IMP. The conduct of first into human studies has come under increased scrutiny following well publicised severe adverse effects experienced by patients enrolled in a trial of TGN1412 in the UK in 2006. Subsequent Phase 1 studies will investigate multiple dosing and further characterise the safety and pharmacology of the IMP.

As development progresses, the IMP will be tested in patients who have the disease that the medicine will be used to treat. Phase 2 studies use a small number of patients to establish whether the IMP is likely to work (the efficacy of the drug), and at what dose. As the IMP progresses to Phase 3 trials, it will be given to an increasing number of patients to gain a more complete picture of its therapeutic and adverse effects.

Many drugs fail to make it through the different stages of testing and do not become medicines. If a medicine does successfully reach the market, monitoring and testing in wider patient populations (post-marketing Phase 4 studies) will help to further assess its effectiveness and safety. In the UK, the process for licensing and monitoring medicines has been overseen and regulated by the European Medicines Agency, and the UK's Medicines and Healthcare products Regulatory Agency (MHRA). These organisations are responsible for ensuring that the medicines that are available for human use in the European Union and UK are safe, effective and good quality. If a medicine does not have the appropriate marketing authorisation, its safety, quality and efficacy cannot be guaranteed.

Influenza vaccine production

In the letter above, Mr Atkins has been invited for a flu (influenza) vaccine. The principle of vaccination is to prompt the body's immune system to respond to a specific infection, such as one or more of the influenza virus types, to reduce the risk of future infection. If it took ten years to bring an influenza vaccine to market, the type of influenza virus present in the population may have changed over that time, and the vaccine would not be effective. In order to address this, influenza vaccines are initially licensed in the usual way. However, each year, manufacturers submit an application to vary the strain of the vaccine, which is reviewed within a much-reduced timescale (approximately eight weeks). This allows the strain of the vaccine to be changed, but not any other properties of the vaccine.

There are also other circumstances in which a medicine can sometimes be approved for use more quickly. The MHRA has an Early Access to Medicines Scheme (EAMS), which allows medicines to be used before they have received full marketing authorisation. This only applies to medicines that will be used for patients with particularly severe conditions where no other treatment options are available. Further information can be found on the MHRA website (www.gov.uk/guidance/apply-for-the-early-access-to-medicines-scheme-eams).

Activity 2.4   Reflection

Take a look at either a paper or electronic copy of the BNF and make some notes on Barrie's medication as detailed at the beginning of this chapter, listing the following:

1. What the medicines are being used to treat – their indication(s).
2. What are the usual doses? Please note these may change from time to time and will be changed according to evidence.
3. What side effects Barrie may encounter.

Barrie tells you he has bought sildenafil for erectile dysfunction from the internet. What would you advise him? Think about the medicine itself, as well as whether it is appropriate for Barrie.

Activity 2.5   Evidence-based practice and research

Drug action table: Use the BNF to complete the following table comparing different products:

Product	Medicinal product (y/n)	What is it used for?	What is its action?
Centrum Advance®			
Fluenz Tetra®			
Levothyroxine			
Enalapril			
Venlafaxine			
Salbutamol			

Figure 2.7   Drug action table

An outline answer is given at the end of this chapter.

Homoeopathic remedies

Case study

Tom's medicines

The medicines administration chart below shows the medicines taken by a patient (Tom). The form is like Barrie's, but Tom has presented for a review of his medication that relates to his arthritic pain. Scanning the list and finding paracetamol implies

(Continued)

(Continued)

Tom uses medication for pain of some description. The list of medicines taken by Tom includes two licensed medicinal products (paracetamol and naproxen) and two homoeopathic remedies (Hypericum and Belladonna).

Medicines to be given regularly				Dose	
1 Date 27/5/22	Drug and form Paracetamol tablet		Route Oral	1g	breakfast
				1g	lunch
Prescriber's signature Dr RSY	Other directions			1g	teatime
				1g	night
2 Date 27/5/22	Drug and form Naproxen tablet		Route Oral	250mg	breakfast
					lunch
Prescriber's signature Dr RSY	Other directions				teatime
				250mg	night
3 Date 27/5/22	Drug and form Hypericum 30c		Route Oral	One	breakfast
					lunch
Prescriber's signature Dr RSY	Other directions Patient's own				teatime
					night
4 Date 27/5/22	Drug and form Belladonna 200c		Route Oral	One	breakfast
					lunch
Prescriber's signature Dr RSY	Other directions Patient's own				teatime
					night

Figure 2.8 Tom's medicine chart

Tom is taking two homoeopathic remedies, Hypericum and Belladonna. Homoeopathy is a system of treating a patient with single or sets of highly diluted substances, which are mainly administered in the form of small tablets. Based on symptoms, a homoeopathic practitioner will attempt to match the most appropriate homoeopathic remedy to the symptoms exhibited by, and characteristics of, each individual patient.

The regulation of Homoeopathic remedies in the UK

There are two schemes that regulate homoeopathic products in the UK. The Simplified Scheme allows a manufacturer to submit data on the quality of their homoeopathic product. To qualify for registration under the Simplified Scheme, homoeopathic products must be for oral or external use only, must be sufficiently diluted to guarantee the safety of the patient and must make no therapeutic claims – contrast this with a medicinal product licence. Under the second scheme, the National Rules Scheme, a homoeopathic manufacturer can claim that the product is used within the homoeopathic tradition for the relief of, or treatment of, minor symptoms and conditions that do not require the supervision of a medical doctor. Note there is no requirement for a homoeopathic product to demonstrate efficacy in order to be registered under this scheme.

The National Institute for Health and Care Excellence (NICE) do not recommend homoeopathy for a number of conditions, due to lack of proven efficacy. These include Otitis media with effusion in under 12s: surgery [CG60], inducing labour [CG70], hyperbilirubinaemia [CG98], Lower Urinary Tract symptoms in men [CG97] and atopic eczema [CG57].

Chapter summary

Despite appearing to be similar, there are some significant differences between the classification and uses of licensed medicinal products, supplements and herbal and homoeopathic products. Medicinal products are licensed on the three key principles of safety, quality and efficacy. The development process for medicines is long and complex, and is designed to provide evidence of safety, quality and efficacy. Summaries of the data generated by this process can be found in the SmPC and BNF, and guides healthcare professionals in the use of these medicines.

Different drugs work in different ways, even if they are achieving the same outcome (such as Harry's antihypertensives). Many drugs act by interfering or hijacking of the body's own control systems, which can be achieved through a variety of different mechanisms. However, one common mechanism is the stimulation or blockade of receptors using agonists or antagonists respectively. Another common mechanism is the inhibition of enzymes, thereby preventing the production or destruction of a variety of substances within the body. Transport proteins and ion channels are essential features of cellular anatomy, which facilitate the movement of substances into and out of the cell. The movement of substances such as ions, and neurotransmitters are essential to the function of many cellular, tissue and organ processes. Inhibiting or activating these transporters and channels can therefore enhance or inhibit specific functions and processes within the body.

Patients choose to access medicines in different ways. This may or may not involve a healthcare professional. However, medicines purchased without medical advice may pose a risk to the patient, due to both clinical and quality reasons. Advising patients in a non-judgemental way may help to improve their condition and ensure their safety.

Activities: Brief outline answers

Activity 2.1 Evidence-based practice and research (page 19)

1. Desogestrel is used for contraception.
2. The dose is 75 micrograms once a day.
3. Desogestrel is available in tablet form, as both generic and branded products.

Activity 2.2 Evidence-based practice and research (page 23)

1. Losartan potassium – Angiotensin II receptor antagonist

2. Vardenafil – Phosphodiesterase type-5 enzyme inhibitor

3. Allopurinol – Xanthine oxidase enzyme inhibitor

4. Montelukast – Leukotriene receptor antagonist

It is worth noting that the BNF doesn't always provide the same information for each drug. You may need to use other sources to find what you need, especially if you are looking for pharmacological information.

Activity 2.3 Evidence-based practice and research (page 29)

The treatment summaries sections of the BNF are a useful source of background information about diseases and medicine groups.

The BNF mentions that annual influenza immunisation is strongly recommended for people with the following conditions:

- chronic respiratory disease;
- chronic heart disease;
- chronic liver disease;
- chronic renal disease at stage 3, 4 or 5;
- chronic neurological disease;
- complement disorders;
- diabetes mellitus;
- immunosuppression because of disease (including asplenia or splenic dysfunction) or treatment (including prolonged systemic corticosteroid treatment [for over one month at dose equivalents of prednisolone: adult and child over 20 kg, 20 mg or more daily; child under 20 kg, 1 mg/kg or more daily], and chemotherapy);
- HIV infection (regardless of immune status);
- morbid obesity (BMI of 40 kg/m2 and above).

Activity 2.4 Reflection (page 31)

Ramipril and amlodipine are licensed medicinal products listed in the BNF. They are both used to treat hypertension as well as other cardiac disorders. St John's Wort is mentioned but there is very little information as it is not often prescribed. However, it is known to affect the way in which certain other medicines work when used together (known as a drug–drug interaction). This is an important consideration when managing all medicines. The Centrum Men® product is an over the counter (OTC) food supplement and therefore will not be listed in the BNF. Both Ramipril and amlodipine can cause erectile dysfunction as a side effect. The sildenafil that Barrie has bought from the internet is used to treat erectile dysfunction. However, the BNF states that a side effect of sildenafil is hypertension, so this may not be a suitable medicine for Barrie. If Ramipril or amlodipine are the cause of Barrie's erectile dysfunction, these may need to be reviewed. Sildenafil may also be abused, and because of this, it is one of the most commonly counterfeited medicines. The quality and safety of the product purchased by Barrie cannot be guaranteed.

Activity 2.5 Evidence-based practice and research (page 31)

Use the BNF to complete the following table comparing different products:

Product	Medicinal product (y/n)	What is it used for?	What is its action?
Centrum®	n	Vitamin Supplement	N/A
Fluenz Tetra®	y	Immunisation against influenza	Immunological
Levothyroxine	y	Hypothyroidism	Replacement
Enalapril	y	Heart failure, hypertension	Enzyme inhibitor
Venlafaxine	y	Depression, anxiety	Transport protein inhibitor
Salbutamol	y	Asthma, reversible airways obstruction	Receptor agonist

Further reading

Aronson JK, Ferner RE (2017) Unlicensed and off-label uses of medicines: definitions and clarification of terminology. Br J Clin Pharmacol. 83: 2615–25.

A review of medicines classification and terminology.

Ashelford S, Raynsford J, Taylor V (2019) Pathophysiology and Pharmacology in Nursing. Second Edition. SAGE.

An introduction to Pharmacology and Physiology for nursing students.

Useful websites

Electronic Medicines Compendium. Available at:

www.medicines.org.uk/emc

Medicines and Healthcare products Regulatory Agency. Available at: www.gov.uk/government/organisations/medicines-and-healthcare-products-regulatory-agency

Chapter 3 Legal and ethical considerations in medicines management

NMC Future Nurse: Standards of Proficiency for Registered Nurses

This chapter will address the following platforms and proficiencies:

Platform 1: Being an accountable professional

At the point of registration, the registered nurse will be able to:

1.9 understand the need to base all decisions regarding care and interventions on people's needs and preferences, recognising and addressing any personal and external factors that may unduly influence their decisions.

1.14 provide and promote non-discriminatory, person centred and sensitive care at all times, reflecting on people's values and beliefs, diverse backgrounds, cultural characteristics, language requirements, needs and preferences, taking account of any need for adjustments.

Platform 3: Assessing needs and planning care

At the point of registration, the registered nurse will be able to:

3.4 understand and apply a person-centred approach to nursing care, demonstrating shared assessment, planning, decision making and goal setting when working with people, their families, communities and populations of all ages.

3.6 effectively assess a person's capacity to make decisions about their own care and to give or withhold consent.

3.8 understand and apply the relevant laws about mental capacity for the country in which you are practising when making decisions in relation to people who do not have capacity.

Platform 4: Providing and evaluating care

At the point of registration, the registered nurse will be able to:

4.2   work in partnership with people to encourage shared decision making in order to support individuals, their families and carers to manage their own care when appropriate.

4.16   demonstrate knowledge of how prescriptions can be generated, the role of generic, unlicensed, and off-label prescribing and an understanding of the potential risks associated with these approaches to prescribing.

Annexe B: Nursing procedures

Part 2: Procedures for the planning, provision and management of person-centred nursing care

11.   Procedural competencies required for best practice, evidence-based medicines administration and optimisation.

11.2   recognise the various procedural routes under which medicines can be prescribed, supplied, dispensed and administered; and the laws, policies, regulations and guidance that underpin them.

11.11 undertake safe storage, transportation and disposal of medicinal products.

Chapter aims

By the end of this chapter you should be able to:

1.   Identify how drugs are classified and how this affects their supply, and storage.
2.   Describe the importance of capacity and consent when managing medicines.
3.   Evaluate the needs of service users, considering their personal, cultural and religious needs when managing their medicines.

Introduction

This chapter explores some of the legal and ethical considerations related to medicines management. These include the principles that underpin the supply of medicines to service users, the storage of medicines prior to administration, and the administration itself. It will illustrate that this needs to be clearly understood in order for the nurse to safely manage medicines in contemporary healthcare. Other important aspects such as capacity, consent and cultural issues that influence medicines use from both the healthcare provider and service user perspective will be discussed. Key pieces of legislation are the Human Medicines Regulations (2012), the misuse of Drugs Regulations (2001), the Mental Health Act (1983) and the Mental Capacity Act (2005).

Definitions

- Prescribing is a process by which a practitioner undertakes appropriate assessment of a patient and develops a treatment plan, which includes decision making around the selection of a medicine.
- Dispensing of a medicine is the process by which a pharmacy takes a prescription and prepares the required medicine for the patient, in order that it can be safely and effectively used.
- The supply of a medicine is a transaction that can include the sale and/or provision of a medicine to a patient for administration to that patient.
- Medicines administration is an act in which a single dose of a prescribed medicine is given to a patient by an authorised person.

Obtaining medicines

In the UK, medicines fall into one of three legal categories, namely: General Sales List medicines (GSL), Pharmacy medicines (P) and Prescription Only Medicines (POM). In addition to the above categories, some medicines are classified as Controlled Drugs (CDs). These have the potential to be misused and are subject to certain restrictions governing their use. The three categories influence how medicines are obtained, stored and administered. GSL medicines are medicines that can be purchased over the counter without requiring healthcare intervention. Pharmacy medicines, also known as P medicines, can only be purchased from registered pharmacies with appropriate pharmacy staff present to supervise the sale. POMs are generally only available after obtaining a prescription from an appropriate practitioner.

Purchasing medicines

A significant number of transactions involving medicines in the UK are purchases made by patients and service users. Individuals can walk into shops and pharmacies to obtain medicines without the need for support or advice from a healthcare professional. For example, a patient can purchase a pack of paracetamol from a local corner store for the treatment of a headache. The medicines that we consider in this context are relatively safe if taken according to their instructions. The legal framework governing medicines use (Human Medicines Regulations, 2012) lists medicines suitable for self-treatment (known as General Sales List (GSL) medicines).

For some drugs, the medicine formulation (including strength, and pack size) will determine its legal category. Therefore, a drug may be a GSL medicine, a P medicine, a POM or a Controlled Drug depending upon these factors. For example, a pack of 100 paracetamol 500mg tablets is a POM, a pack of ten paracetamol 80mg suppositories is a P medicine, and a pack of 16 paracetamol 500mg tablets is a GSL medicine.

Supplying medicines: Prescribing, dispensing and ward supply

Medicines that are more complex to manage require the intervention of healthcare professionals, and greater governance in their supply. Several mechanisms are used to supply such medicines. One of the most common is obtaining a prescription (for example from a GP or practice nurse) and its dispensing from a community pharmacy. This is the typical way in which POMs are supplied, although supplies of other medicines may also sometimes be made by prescription. For a prescription to be legal, it must meet the requirements outlined in the Human Medicines Regulations, with additional requirements applying to prescriptions for Controlled Drugs.

The principles and practice of medicines transactions are governed by the same legal requirements in the community or hospital setting. However, you will notice differences relating to governance, paperwork and procedures. Compare the chart Adeola is using for administration in a ward setting (Figure 3.1) with the community-based prescription (Figure 3.2) illustrated below. The legal frameworks that govern prescribing are the same, but the process and governance would be different.

In secondary care settings, prescribers make clinical decisions regarding medicines and the inpatient chart or a prescription is used to obtain the medicine, which is supplied or administered to the patient. Medicines are usually ordered from a hospital pharmacy department, dispensed, and then supplied to the ward as stock or for an individual patient. Typically, in a hospital setting, all of the patient's medicines (whether GSL, P or POM) will be written on the inpatient chart in order to facilitate supply and administration.

One notable difference between the supply of medicines in the community and hospital settings relates to Controlled Drugs. In a hospital inpatient ward, Controlled Drugs are often ordered via a specific requisition (rather than a prescription for an individual patient), which is dispensed by the pharmacy. This helps to monitor the supply of these potentially dangerous and misused medicines. The Misuse of Drugs Regulations 2001 groups Controlled Drugs into different 'Schedules' according to their level of perceived risk. Schedule 1 drugs cannot be legally obtained without a Home Office licence and are perceived to have no therapeutic value. Controlled Drugs used in clinical practice are grouped into schedules 2, 3, 4 and 5, with reducing levels of associated regulation. Practice may vary slightly between hospitals, so local policies should be followed. However, medicines in Schedule 2 (e.g. amfetamine, and strong opioids) and schedule 3 (e.g. barbiturates, temazepam, tramadol) are typically obtained via a specific requisition, and stored in a separate cupboard. Medicines in schedule 5 are subject to the least restrictions, and in some cases may be available to purchase as P medicines from pharmacies. One example is a pack of 12 dihydrocodeine with paracetamol 7.46mg/500mg tablets.

Case study

Adeola's 'drug round'

Adeola is a student nurse who is undertaking a practice placement in a ward setting. She is going to assist with a medicines administration round ('drug round') and sees the chart illustrated in Figure 3.1. She reviews the chart before the round and starts to familiarise herself with the medicines. Usually she sees one prescriber's signature on the chart (she assumed they were a doctor who worked on the ward) but notices that the 'Prescriber's signature' boxes also include those of a pharmacist and a nurse. Adeola speaks to her mentor about the different signatures, as she was unfamiliar with the idea of nurses and pharmacists prescribing medicines.

Activity 3.1 Evidence-based practice

Visit the Pharmaceutical Services Negotiating Committee website and look at the page 'Who can prescribe what, available at: https://psnc.org.uk/dispensing-supply/receiving-a-prescription/who-can-prescribe-what/. This page outlines the healthcare professionals

Medicines to be given regularly				Dose	
1 Date 27/5/22	Drug and form Morphine sulphate tablet		Route Oral	10mg	breakfast
				10mg	lunch
Prescriber's signature Dr RSY	Other directions			10mg	teatime
				10mg	night
2 Date 27/5/22	Drug and form Cyclizine tablet		Route Oral	50mg	breakfast
				50mg	lunch
Prescriber's signature Dr RSY	Other directions				teatime
				50mg	night
3 Date 27/5/22	Drug and form Senna tablet		Route Oral		breakfast
					lunch
Prescriber's signature PND (Pharmacist)	Other directions				teatime
				15mg	night
4 Date 27/5/22	Drug and form Levothyroxine sodium		Route Oral	25 micrograms	breakfast
					lunch
Prescriber's signature BDP (Senior nurse)	Other directions				teatime
					night

Figure 3.1 Inpatient medicine chart for Adeola's medicine administration round ('drug' round)

who can prescribe, and what differences there may be between the prescribing rights of each profession. In Figure 3.1, you can see that a doctor, a pharmacist and a nurse have all prescribed medicines. Use the information on the website to identify whether these practitioners can prescribe the medicines indicated.

An outline answer is given at the end of this chapter.

Healthcare professionals with prescribing rights

In the UK, the doctor is typically the most frequent prescriber of medicines. However, the prescribing landscape in the UK is changing, with an increasing number of prescribers who do not have medical training, sometimes known as non-medical prescribers. The term 'appropriate practitioner' is now used to describe those who can prescribe. In addition to doctors and dentists, the list of 'appropriate practitioners' currently includes nurses, midwives, paramedics, pharmacists, physiotherapists, radiographers and dieticians, who have a range of prescribing roles that fit with their sphere of practice and their professional competence. These prescribers are known as independent prescribers and are responsible for the assessment, diagnosis and clinical management of a patient and the appropriate use of medicines in that context.

As well as independent prescribing, non-medical prescribers can also prescribe medicines through a mechanism known as supplementary prescribing. Supplementary prescribing is a voluntary partnership between an independent prescriber (who is a doctor or a dentist) and a supplementary prescriber (such as a nurse), to implement an agreed clinical management plan (CMP) for an individual patient. The independent prescriber retains responsibility for diagnosing the condition to be treated. However, the CMP outlines the approach for ongoing management, which is undertaken by the supplementary prescriber. Supplementary prescribing was essentially a stage in the progression of non-medical healthcare professionals to full independent prescribing. It is still utilised occasionally, although most prescribing decisions, such as those illustrated on the inpatient chart in Figure 3.1, are reached through independent prescribing.

Healthcare professionals, whether they are medical or non-medical, will prescribe within their own area of competence. A prescriber who works in oncology will primarily prescribe oncological medicines and other medicines required to holistically manage a patient in that setting. The oncology practitioner will very rarely make a treatment decision outside their scope of practice. For example, oncological practitioners will not diagnose and prescribe medicines to treat schizophrenia.

Supplying Prescription Only Medicines without a prescription

There are a number of ways that Prescription Only Medicines can be sold or supplied without needing a prescription. The following sections give examples of these and explain the context in which they may be used.

Patient specific directions

A patient specific direction (PSD) is accepted to mean a written instruction, typically from a prescriber, for a medicine to be supplied or administered to a named patient after the prescriber has assessed that patient on an individual basis. The law in the UK does not define a PSD. In hospitals, written PSDs are encountered as inpatient charts similar to that seen by Adeola. Legally there is no stipulation as to exactly what should be included on a PSD, but there must be enough information available for those using the PSD to safely administer the supplied medicine. In a hospital setting when a patient is ready to be discharged, information from the hospital inpatient chart is typically transcribed onto an order form for the hospital pharmacy to prepare a supply of medicines to take home. This process is known as transcribing and is not the same as prescribing.

Patient group direction

A patient group direction (PGD) is defined in the Human Medicines Regulations (2012) as a written direction that facilitates the supply and/or administration of a specified medicine or medicines, by named authorised health professionals, to a specified group of patients, for treatment of a specific condition. PGDs are commonly used in vaccination clinics and sexual health clinics to enable the supply and administration of medicines in a defined and controlled manner. PGDs are usually developed after careful consideration of all of the potential ways in which the medicine could be supplied or administered to patients or service users, including the availability and practicality of prescribing. PGDs expedite patient care without the need for the prescribing interaction, but without compromising the safety of the service user.

Obtaining medicines in an emergency

Prescription Only Medicines (POM) can be supplied without a prescription in emergencies, if certain conditions are met. A pharmacist, for example, may supply a POM to a patient without a prescription. Take the example of a service user who goes on holiday and forgets their asthma inhaler and who is unable to get access to medical support and therefore a prescription. A pharmacist (following a set of criteria and instructions) would be able to supply the medicine to the service user.

Medicines such as oxygen and adrenaline (epinephrine) and other medicines used to save lives can be administered and supplied without a prescription in emergency situations. The law in the UK also allows a relaxation of the requirements for the emergency supply of medicines in a pandemic or an imminent pandemic which is declared by the appropriate government departments.

Principles of medicines storage

Medicines are stored in different ways for a number of reasons such as their chemical nature, their likelihood of deterioration, legal requirements and safe medicine management principles. The following section explores some of these factors in more detail.

Case study   (continued)

Adeola's 'drug round'

Adeola recalls seeing some of the medicines needed for her patient in the ward stock cupboard, the medicines trolley and in the patient's own medicines locker. However, she doesn't recall seeing the morphine. She asks her mentor where the morphine is stored, and the mentor explains that it is locked in the Controlled Drugs (CD) cupboard. This prompts a discussion about how Adeola will be responsible for obtaining and storing medicines when she is qualified. The text below explains some of the key factors that determine where and how medicines are stored.

Activity 3.2   Evidence-based practice and research

Look again at the medicine chart in Figure 3.1. Using the BNF look up each medicine, and as far as possible, identify whether it is a controlled drug. You should be able to find this information in the drug monograph.

An outline answer is given at the end of this chapter.

Chemical composition and prevention of deterioration

Medicines, like foodstuffs and other chemicals, are subject to deterioration, and a number of factors influence the rate of deterioration, including how the medicine is stored. The main method of protecting against deterioration is appropriate packaging and storage (e.g. keeping the medicine in its original blister pack) in an appropriate physical setting. This protects the medicine from factors such as moisture, exposure to oxygen in the air, light and inappropriate temperature, which can affect its stability and efficacy. Total Parenteral Nutrition products, when they are reconstituted for administration, are sensitive to light and will deteriorate if exposed to light for extended periods.

A number of medicines are stored in a refrigerator. In clinical settings, refrigerators are maintained and monitored carefully to ensure that they sustain a given temperature, usually between 4 and 8°c. Medicines such as insulin should not be allowed to freeze or be exposed to heat, in order to ensure their pharmacological efficacy.

Legal classification

In hospital environments, medicines of all types are stored in locked areas, e.g. patients' own medicine lockers, large storage cupboards and 'drug trolleys'. In addition, a number of controlled drugs are subject to additional safe storage requirements as specified in the Misuse of Drugs Regulations (2001). Controlled drugs in Schedule 2 and some of those in Schedule 3 must be stored in specific locked cupboards. Records of the quantities of these medicines obtained and administered are required due to their potential for misuse. As with the ordering of medicines, local policies may be in place relating to specific storage requirements, and these should always be followed.

Medicine storage is dictated by the nature of the care environment

In a patient's home, there are no legal requirements as to how medicines should be stored. However, medicines should be stored in a cool, dry and secure place. This environment maintains the stability of the medicine and helps to maintain its quality and effectiveness. Medicines should be stored out of the reach of children and consideration should be given to the storage of drugs that are liable to misuse (for example morphine and other opioids), to prevent them falling into the wrong hands and to prevent accidental overdose. The number of appropriate locations available in the home is limited in comparison to the secondary care context. For example, medicines such as insulin may be found stored alongside food in the refrigerator in a patient's home – this would not be acceptable in a clinical setting. Within other residential care facilities such as nursing homes, the storage of medicines may vary depending on the capacity and level of independence of the patients in question.

Case study

Adeola's community placement

In Adeola's next placement, she is spending some time with the district nursing team and visiting a patient who is receiving morphine at home. She recalls the process and paperwork required to acquire the morphine in the ward setting and asks about the process of obtaining morphine as they cannot recall a CD cupboard at the District Nursing base. Adeola's mentor, Raj, a district nursing team lead, explains that the morphine is with the patient and they will be using the morphine from the patient's own supply.

Activity 3.3 Reflection

Figure 3.2 is an illustration of an FP10 type (community) prescription for MXL (a capsule containing morphine) for a patient. Compare and contrast the prescription with the ward chart studied earlier.

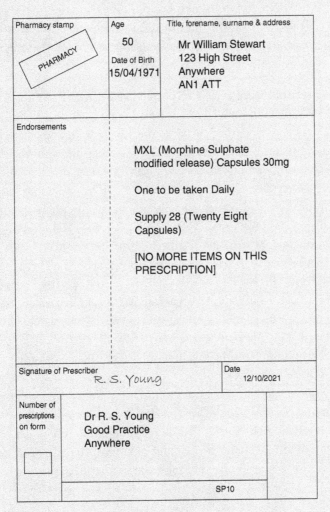

Pharmacy stamp	Age	Title, forename, surname & address
PHARMACY	50	Mr William Stewart
	Date of Birth	123 High Street
	15/04/1971	Anywhere
		AN1 ATT

Endorsements

MXL (Morphine Sulphate modified release) Capsules 30mg

One to be taken Daily

Supply 28 (Twenty Eight Capsules)

[NO MORE ITEMS ON THIS PRESCRIPTION]

Signature of Prescriber
R. S. Young

Date
12/10/2021

Number of prescriptions on form

Dr R. S. Young
Good Practice
Anywhere

SP10

Figure 3.2 **Prescription for community pharmacy dispensing**

An outline answer is given at the end of this chapter.

Legal, ethical and cultural factors to consider when administering medicines

The next part of this chapter explores some of the patient-centred factors that need to be considered when administering medicines. Although the focus is on administration, these may also be applicable to your wider role in managing medicines.

Activity 3.4   Reflection

The three scenarios below give some examples of people refusing to take the medicine that has been recommended or prescribed for them, and which you might encounter in your practice. Read the scenarios and reflect upon how you might manage each situation. Would you do the same thing in each case, or does each scenario require a different approach? The text in the following section of the chapter will explore these scenarios and provide guidance of the approach that might be taken in each case.

1. Arwel is a 35-year-old man, who is in hospital recovering from a successful surgical procedure. He is otherwise well and has no ongoing medical conditions. For the last 24 hours he has been prescribed the antibiotic flucloxacillin, to be given via the intravenous route four times a day. He finds the injection uncomfortable, and tells the nurse looking after him that he doesn't want to have it anymore. Arwel has recovered well from the surgery and is able to swallow, so asks if he could have the flucloxacillin orally (as capsules) instead. The nurse tells him that he must have the injection as that is what the doctor has prescribed.

2. Claire is a 71-year-old woman, and is suffering from moderately severe dementia. She is living in a care home and has become increasingly confused over the last few days. She does not know where she is, or why she is there, and says that she wants to go back home to live with her husband, who passed away several years ago. She is seen by a nurse practitioner from the local GP surgery, who diagnoses an acute lower urinary tract infection (UTI). The nurse explains to Claire that she will need to take the antibiotic nitrofurantoin to treat the infection. Claire says that she doesn't want to take it; she just wants to go home.

3. Priti is a 42-year-old woman, diagnosed with schizophrenia, who is currently detained in hospital under Section 3 of the Mental Health Act. She is acutely unwell with delusions about her neighbour, saying that he is spying on her on behalf of the CIA. She is prescribed the antipsychotic risperidone to control her psychotic symptoms, and beclometasone for asthma, but is refusing to take either of them.

An outline answer is given at the end of this chapter.

Before any treatment can be given (or any test or examination undertaken), the patient must give their consent or permission. In each of the scenarios above, the person is not willing to take the medicine recommended for them and is therefore not consenting to treatment. However, this does not mean that you can manage each scenario in the same way. There are different legal and ethical factors to consider when helping people to make decisions about the management of their medicines. In addition to the need for people to consent to treatment, you may also need to think about the Mental Capacity Act and in some cases the Mental Health Act.

Consent to treatment

For a person to give valid consent to treatment:

- they must be told (or informed) about what the treatment involves;
- they must have the ability (or capacity) to make the decision;
- they must give the consent voluntarily.

In the first scenario, Arwel is recovering from surgery, but appears to be otherwise well. There is nothing to suggest that he has a condition such as a mental illness, or brain injury that would make him unable to make decisions for himself. Furthermore, he has made the request to change to an oral medicine of his own choice and does not appear to have been pressured or coerced into doing so. Therefore, it appears that two out of the three criteria above have been met. However, is Arwel making an informed decision? Without knowing what he has been told about his treatment we cannot be sure.

To make an informed decision, a person must understand what is involved with the treatment, what are the benefits and risks, and what the alternatives are, including what would happen if nothing were done. When providing the information, it should be patient focused, and not restricted to what you as a healthcare professional think they need to know. Ultimately, as a healthcare professional, you should work together with your patient, ensure they have the information that they want, and try to come to a shared decision on the best way forward to meet their needs.

After surgery, Arwel would have been prescribed an antibiotic to reduce his risk of developing an infection. The intravenous route allows administration of a medicine to patients who might be unconscious or unable to swallow. Medicines given intravenously also tend to be more effective than those given orally. Therefore, by requesting a change to oral flucloxacillin, Arwel might be requesting a form of the medicine that is less effective, which might increase his chance of experiencing an infection. However, whilst this decision might seem inappropriate or ill-advised, it does not mean that the request should be ignored. If Arwel has been informed of, and understands the risks, and meets the other criteria for making an informed choice, his decision should be respected, and where possible, a shared decision regarding his treatment made. If a patient requests a treatment that would provide no benefit and a shared decision cannot be reached, the healthcare professional is not obliged to pursue the requested course of action, but should explain that the patient is able to pursue other options including seeking a second opinion.

The Mental Capacity Act

Part of the criteria that determines whether someone can give informed consent requires the person to have capacity to make decisions. According to the 2005 Mental Capacity Act, in order to have capacity, the person must be able to understand the information they have been given, retain the information, and use it to make the decision. In certain circumstances, a person may lack capacity due to illness or injury.

In the second scenario, Claire has dementia, a disorder that affects memory, as well as someone's ability to understand and process information (sometimes known as their cognitive function). This, along with other conditions such as learning disability, brain injury and stroke, can limit a person's capacity to make certain decisions. However, whilst these conditions might affect cognitive function and capacity, a person should be assumed to have capacity unless it can be proved otherwise. Due to her dementia, Claire may lack capacity to make an informed choice about the antibiotic needed to treat her UTI. She therefore requires an assessment of her capacity to make this decision, based upon her ability to understand, retain and use the information needed to make the decision. If the assessment indicates that Claire has capacity, as in the first scenario, if a shared decision cannot be reached, her wish to refuse the antibiotic treatment should be respected, even if it appears unwise.

If an assessment indicates that Claire lacks capacity to make a decision about her antibiotic, a number of options may need to be considered.

Firstly, if the treatment is not urgent, Claire's capacity could be re-assessed at a future time or date. Capacity can fluctuate, and it is possible that Claire will regain capacity in the future. Similarly, it may be possible to present the information in a different way or ask a family member or carer to explain the information, which might make Claire feel more comfortable and better able to make the decision. It should also be noted that whilst Claire may not have capacity to make a decision regarding her medicine, she may have capacity to make other decisions, for example whether to have a bath.

Secondly, Claire may have made an Advance Decision (a legally binding statement about her future wishes), also known as a living will. An Advance Decision is made whilst a person still has capacity and outlines their wish to refuse certain treatments should they lose capacity in the future. It applies to specific treatments, so if Claire has made an Advance Decision, it would have to state that she did not wish to receive antibiotics to be valid in this situation.

Thirdly, Claire may have granted Lasting Power of Attorney (LPA) for health and welfare to someone, allowing them to make decisions about her treatment on her behalf. As with an Advance Decision, LPA is granted whilst the person still has capacity, and can be used if capacity is lost at some point in the future. The decisions made by the attorney must be in the person's best interests, taking into account what they would have wanted if they still had capacity.

If Claire lacks capacity, and none of the above applies, a decision must be made in her best interests by the treating team. When deciding on the appropriate course of action, the team should consider what Claire would have wanted based on her known beliefs and wishes, and what would be the least restrictive option. The team should also consult with family members or carers and try to include Claire in the process. More information about making decisions in someone's best interests can be found in the Mental Capacity Act 2005 Code of Practice.

The Mental Health Act

The final scenario given in Activity 3.4 considers Priti, who is detained in hospital under section 3 of the 1983 Mental Health Act. The Mental Health Act is the legislation governing the assessment, care and treatment of people with mental illnesses.

Due to the symptoms of her mental illness, Priti may not have capacity to make a decision regarding her treatment. However, even if she did have capacity, she may not be in a position to refuse treatment. This is because if the treating clinician considers it necessary, patients detained under certain sections of the Mental Health Act can be given treatment for their mental illness, even if they have capacity to refuse. Priti is detained under section 3 of the Mental Health Act, and treatment can be given whether she consents or not. Depending upon the length of time that she has been detained, certain conditions may apply. More information can be found in the Mental Health Act 1983: Code of Practice.

In this scenario, Priti was also refusing to take beclometasone. Although the Mental Health Act allows treatments for mental illness to be administered against a patient's wishes, this does not apply to treatments for physical illness. Medicines for physical illnesses cannot be given if the patient has capacity to refuse them, even if the decision appears unwise or might result in harm. Therefore, if Priti had capacity she could refuse beclomethasone, which is for the management of her asthma.

Cultural aspects

The previous examples have discussed some of the legal frameworks influencing medicines management. However, cultural and ethical considerations are also important, and some of these aspects are described in the following section.

Case study

Name:	Abdul Sala		DOB: 23/4/1964	
Condition(s):	Chest infection			
Medicine	Formulation/route	Dose	Frequency	
Cefalexin	Capsule	250mg	Every 6 hours	

Figure 3.3 Abdul's medicine

(Continued)

(Continued)

Abdul is a 52-year-old estate agent in generally good health, with no ongoing chronic diseases or health concerns. However, he has developed a chest infection, for which his GP prescribes antibiotics. Abdul has been instructed to take his antibiotic four times a day (every six hours), however, it is currently Ramadan and he does not want to swallow any medicine during daylight hours. It will not be possible to take the medicine at the times required and maintain his daytime fast. Abdul is also concerned that the capsules are made of gelatin; if this is made from pork or beef then it may not be Halal, which would also go against his beliefs.

Abdul asks for your advice about taking his antibiotics. What would you tell him?

Adjusting treatments to meet the individual cultural or religious needs of patients

Abdul's concerns relate to being unable to take the prescribed medicine at the recommended timings. But why are drug doses timed the way that they are; why don't we take every drug just once per day?

Different drugs are cleared from the body at different rates. The faster the drug is cleared, the more frequently it will have to be dosed. If the doses are too far apart the levels of drug in the body will drop and it will cease to be effective. In Abdul's case this could mean the drug being ineffective for treating his infection. If the doses of the drug are administered too closely together, then the drug can accumulate in the body and reach toxic levels. The ideal spacing of doses should keep the levels of drug in the body at a 'steady state' by balancing the rate of drug entering the body with the rate of it leaving.

Abdul believes that to consume the antibiotics during daylight hours would mean breaking his Ramadan fast. He feels that he faces the choice of either following the tenets of his beliefs or receiving proper treatment for his infection. It can be easy for healthcare professionals to focus on the treatment of ill health as the number one priority and dismiss other concerns. However, it is always important to remember that we must respect people's choices and work to find solutions that allow appropriate treatment whilst allowing them to hold true to their beliefs.

One solution might be to find an alternative treatment that can be dosed less often. However, this may not be possible as alternate antibiotics may not be effective. Another solution might be to change the dosing strategy of Abdul's antibiotic. The BNF states that cefalexin can be dosed as 500mg every 12 hours. This would result in Abdul receiving 1g every 24 hours but would allow Abdul to take the required medicine whilst respecting his fast. This adjustment of dosing will solve Abdul's problem in this circumstance, but is not always possible. With many drugs, taking higher doses less often is not a viable course of action, as the higher doses may result in toxicity.

Abdul's second query is about the possibility of the medicine containing pork gelatin. At first this may seem like an odd question; why would there be pork in cefalexin? However, it is important to remember that a medicine is more than just the drug. The drug is the active ingredient, but this is only part of what you take. The drug may be dissolved in a fluid, contained within a tablet of lactose or as in this case, contained within a capsule made of gelatin. Medicines may also be coloured with food dyes, have added preservatives or other agents intended to extend the storage life of the drug or make it more palatable or easy to swallow. These other ingredients are referred to as 'excipients'. A full list of a medicine's excipients can usually be found on the patient information leaflet or in the Summary of Product Characteristics (SmPC). When considering the safe administration of medicines, it is important to consider not only the active ingredient of a medicine but also its excipients. A patient may have no issues with the drug, but it is quite possible for a patient to have an allergy, intolerance or other objection to an excipient.

In this case study the patient's concern relates to the presence of the excipient gelatin within the medicine formulation. This is not an isolated or unusual challenge and may need to be considered for a notable cross-section of our society. Many medicines contain or are derived from animal products such as gelatin, lactose (derived from milk and often using animal rennet in its extraction) and magnesium stearate (derived from rendered animal fats), which depending on their source may be in conflict with the adherents of various religions such as Judasim, Budhism or Hinduism.

The use of medicines containing animal products may also present a challenge for vegetarians, vegans or others who have concerns over animal welfare. This may extend to the refusal of medicines that use animal products in their manufacture or testing and development (although this is highly unusual).

The solution to this problem may not always be straightforward. For some people, the medical necessity of the treatment may over-rule their moral or religious objections; however, for others it may be necessary to find an alternative treatment. In Abdul's case, as the gelatin is an excipient and not the active ingredient of the medicine, the best option may be to find an alternative formulation of cefalexin that does not contain gelatin.

Activity 3.5   Research

In this section we have considered the importance of considering the excipients of a medicine. However, these will not be included on the drug chart, prescription or even in the BNF. These can usually be found in the Patient information leaflet (PIL) which is included

(Continued)

(Continued)

in the medicine packaging or in the Summary of Product Characteristics (SmPC). Many SmPCs for medicines licensed in the UK can be found on the Electronic Medicines Compendium (EMC) website at www.medcines.org.uk.

Go to this website and search for common drugs that you are familiar with. For each drug you may see that there is a different SmPC for each formulation, strength and manufacturer. When you access the SmPC you will see that it is divided into numbered sections. The 'List of excipients' is located in Section 6.1. Look at this for a variety of medicines and consider whether there are any excipients that might present a problem for certain patients.

In the case study above, the concerns related to the presence of gelatin within the cefalexin capsules. Use the EMC to look for alternative formulations of cefalexin that do not contain gelatin.

An outline answer is given at the end of the chapter.

Crushing medicines

Case study

Name:	Glenys Dobson		DOB: 15/6/1935	
Condition(s):	Type 2 diabetes mellitus			
Medicine	Formulation/route	Dose	Frequency	
Metformin (M/R)	Tablet	500mg	Once a day	

Figure 3.4 Glenys's medicine

Glenys has been admitted to a local general hospital for review of her diabetes. When it comes to administering her medicines, she refuses and becomes distressed. Her daughter, who is with her, says that they normally just crush it up and put it in her yoghurt.

This situation raises two significant issues. Firstly, should you crush, break or otherwise alter the formulation of a medicine in order to make it easier to give, and secondly, should you secretly administer a medicine to a patient who has refused it?

There are circumstances where a tablet cannot be easily given; perhaps it tastes bad or the patient has a nasogastric (NG) tube in place. In these circumstances, crushing the tablet or dissolving it in water would seem a simple solution. Some medicines are designed with these options in mind; they are scored for breaking or formulated in such a way that the medicine will dissolve easily in water. In these cases, the medicine's Patient Information Leaflet (PIL) and SmPC will make these options clear. However, if the manufacturer of the medicine has not formulated it with this in mind, it is important to consider that if you interfere with the formulation you create a new unlicensed medicine (as discussed in Chapter 2). This does not prohibit you from using it but does have implications for consent and accountability should things go wrong. As the medicine is being used outside of the manufacturer's recommendations, the patient must be informed so that they can provide informed consent to the use of the medicine in this manner. Furthermore, if the patient suffers a negative outcome, the practitioners who prescribed and administered the medicine could be considered liable.

A further complication is that dissolving or crushing may impede the proper working of the drug or medicine; this is discussed in more depth in Chapter 4. Due to these issues, it is usually better to use a different formulation (such as a syrup or suspension) rather than to crush a tablet. However, there are circumstances where this is not possible and crushing the tablet may be the only means of facilitating the administration of the drug. If a practitioner is presented with this situation, the decision to crush the medicine should not be taken lightly and should be discussed with the prescriber or pharmacist.

Activity 3.6   Research

In the above case study, it is suggested that a tablet might be crushed in order to assist the patient swallowing the medicine. Use the EMC (www.medicines.org.uk) to search for an alternative formulation which could be used to remove the need to crush the tablet. Is there anything else that needs to be considered?

An outline answer is given at the end of the chapter.

Covert administration

The second issue that this case study presents is whether it is acceptable to hide the medicine (whether crushed or not) in the patient's food. This concept essentially means tricking the patient into taking their medicine without their consent and is referred to as 'covert administration'.

At first, the idea of secretly administering a medicine without the patient's consent seems to be in complete contravention of the principle of informed consent. However, in some circumstances it may be an unfortunate necessity. The important question to ask is why Glenys is refusing her tablet. If she understands that it is a medicine, she understands what it is for, and understands what the impact of not taking it might have on her health, then she has the right to refuse it and this should be respected. However, Glenys has dementia, and may not understand what the medicine is, and not like its bitter taste. If this is the case it may be possible to find a more palatable formulation, which Glenys will not refuse. However, if no alternative can be found, consideration of Glenys' capacity may be required, and a decision made to undertake covert administration if it is in her best interests.

The decision to administer medicines covertly should not be taken lightly or independently. The issue should be discussed within the healthcare team and, where possible, the patient's family or carer. The decision to administer drugs covertly should always be made with the best interests of the patient as the primary consideration (rather than convenience for the staff or family). Decisions should be clearly recorded and regularly reviewed.

Case study

Anthony is a 46-year-old patient with bipolar disorder and diabetes, who has been admitted to your medical ward for stabilisation of his blood glucose. As a result of his bipolar disorder, Anthony experiences periodic episodes of elevated mood (mania) and low mood (depression), separated by periods of euthymia (normal mood). His mood is currently euthymic (normal). In addition to his diabetes medicines, he is prescribed lithium (Priadel®) 800mg at night for the treatment of his bipolar disorder. When you give Anthony the lithium tablets for his night-time dose, he refuses to take them. He says that he doesn't like them because they blunt his emotions, even though he knows that they help to prevent the fluctuations in his mood that result in episodes of mania and depression.

Activity 3.7   Reflection

Reflect upon what you have read in this chapter, and decide whether Anthony is able to refuse the lithium treatment for his mental illness whilst he is in hospital, or whether you should enforce the treatment to prevent a relapse of his mental illness.

An outline answer is given at the end of the chapter.

Chapter summary

This chapter has explored some of the legal and ethical considerations relevant to medicines management. The supply and storage of medicines is regulated by the Human Medicines Regulations (2012). The specific requirements for a medicine depend largely upon its legal classification as a GSL, P or POM, and the context of care in which you are working.

In addition to working within the legal requirements of the regulations, it is also important to be familiar with and adhere to local policies specific to your place of work.

When working with patients or service users it is essential to take a patient-centred approach when managing their medicines. This could involve working within relevant legal frameworks to achieve the best outcome. It may also require application of pharmacological and medicine formulation knowledge to identify safe and effective alternative treatment options when the usual approach is not possible. An awareness that a multidisciplinary approach involving the wider healthcare team as well as the patient (and where applicable their carer) is likely to be needed to achieve this is essential.

Activities: Brief outline answers

Activity 3.1 Evidence-based practice (page 40)

There are legally described, profession specific, limitations associated with prescribing. For example, doctors registered in the UK can prescribe a range of controlled drugs, they can prescribe unlicensed medicines and they can authorise the emergency supply of prescription only medicines. In contrast, non-medical prescribers (for example physiotherapists) may have more limited prescribing rights. At the time of writing, a physiotherapist independent prescriber can only prescribe a small range of controlled drugs, they can only prescribe off-label medicines subject to accepted clinical practice (but not unlicensed medicines) and they can authorise emergency supply for only a very limited number of medicines within their sphere of competence. Similarly, there are other subtle differences between prescribing that may be undertaken by other practitioners such as nurses, pharmacists and paramedics. Prescribing for non-medical healthcare professionals has evolved over time and continues to evolve. It is therefore important to check the latest advice relating to the medicines that different non-medical prescribers can prescribe.

Activity 3.2 Evidence-based practice and research (page 43)

The BNF monograph contains information on the legal classification of a medicine in the 'Medicinal Forms' section (typically found at the end of the monograph). The legal classification of a medicine can vary according to the nature of the formulation (including strength and type). It is therefore important to make sure that you are looking up the correct formulation. The legal classification is also subject to change over time, and the most up to date information should always be used.

At the time of writing, the legal classification of the medicines in Figure 2.1 noted in the BNF is:

Morphine tablet: POM (Prescription Only Medicine); CD2 (Controlled Drug Schedule 2)

Cyclizine tablet: P (Pharmacy Medicine)

Senna tablet: P (Pharmacy Medicine)

Levothyroxine tablet: POM (Prescription Only Medicine)

Activity 3.3 Reflection (page 45)

Much of the information found on the inpatient medicine chart and the FP10 prescription for morphine is the same. Both include the name, form and strength of the drug, as well as the dose. Both are signed by the prescriber, and both are dated. The FP10 prescription includes the patient's name and address; this would also be found on the inpatient chart, but is not represented in the extract shown in Figure 2.1. The FP10 prescription also includes the total amount of the medicine to be supplied. As morphine is a Schedule 2 controlled drug, this is specified in both words (Twenty-eight) and numbers (28). This reflects the legal status of the FP10 as a prescription, which allows the medicine to be dispensed by a community pharmacy.

Activity 3.4 Reflection (page 46)

Arwel: Here, the patient appears to have capacity to refuse the medicine prescribed for him, and his opinion should be respected. If the doctor agrees, an oral antibiotic could be prescribed.

Claire: Here, the patient may lack capacity to make a decision about her treatment due to her dementia. An assessment of her capacity is needed. The approach to her management that is taken will depend upon the outcome of the assessment, and where relevant any previous granting of Legal Power of Attorney, advance decision, or a decision made in the patient's best interests.

Priti: Here the patient is detained under section 3 of the Mental Health Act. As a result, even if she is refusing it, treatment for her psychotic illness (risperidone) can be enforced. However, depending upon her circumstances, this may require the opinion of a 'Second Opinion Approved Doctor' who is independent of her care team. As the beclomethasone inhaler is for the treatment of her asthma and not for the treatment of a mental illness, administration cannot be enforced under the Mental Health Act.

Activity 3.5 Research (page 51)

Part 2. There are a variety of formulations for cefalexin available including tablets, which do not contain gelatin. However, they do contain magnesium stearate and lactose (which are also animal derivatives). There is also a liquid formulation, which does not contain these excipients.

Activity 3.6 Research (page 53)

There are a multitude of liquid preparations available for metformin. However, liquid preparations are 'immediate release' and the patient's current prescription is for a modified release capsule. A direct swap would not be possible, and the dosing regimen may need to be altered.

Activity 3.7 Reflection (page 54)

Although Anthony is a hospital inpatient and is refusing the treatment prescribed for his mental health (bipolar) disorder, his lithium cannot be enforced. This is because he is not a detained patient under a section of the Mental Health Act, and he appears to have capacity to make decisions regarding his treatment. His mood is currently euthymic, and he understands what the lithium is for, and what will happen if he doesn't take it. His decision should therefore be respected. If Anthony's mental state deteriorated and he subsequently met the criteria for detention and treatment of his mental illness, under certain sections of the Mental Health Act it would be possible to mandate his lithium.

Further reading

British National Formulary. Medicines Guidance. Controlled Drugs and drug dependence. Available at: https://bnf.nice.org.uk/guidance/controlled-drugs-and-drug-dependence.html

Provides advice on the management of controlled drugs.

Mental Health Act 1983: Code of Practice. Available at: https://assets.publishing.service.gov.uk/government/uploads/system/uploads/attachment_data/file/435512/MHA_Code_of_Practice.PDF

Provides guidance on how the Mental Health Act should be applied in practice.

Mental Capacity Act 2005: Code of Practice. Available at: https://assets.publishing.service.gov.uk/government/uploads/system/uploads/attachment_data/file/921428/Mental-capacity-act-code-of-practice.pdf

Provides guidance on how the Mental Capacity Act should be applied in practice.

National Institute for Health and Care Excellence (NICE). 2014. SC1 Managing medicines in care homes. Available at: www.nice.org.uk/guidance/sc1

Provides guidance on the safe and effective management of medicines in care homes.

Royal Pharmaceutical Society. Professional guidance on the safe and secure handling of medicines. Available at: www.rpharms.com/recognition/setting-professional-standards/safe-and-secure-handling-of-medicines/professional-guidance-on-the-safe-and-secure-handling-of-medicines?welcome=true

Provides advice on the handling of medicines, including obtaining, storing and disposing of medicines.

Useful websites

British National Formulary. Medicines Guidance. Controlled Drugs and drug dependence. Available at: https://bnf.nice.org.uk/guidance/controlled-drugs-and-drug-dependence.html

Royal Pharmaceutical Society. Professional guidance on the safe and secure handling of medicines. Available at: www.rpharms.com/recognition/setting-professional-standards/safe-and-secure-handling-of-medicines/professional-guidance-on-the-safe-and-secure-handling-of-medicines?welcome=true

Mental Health Act 1983: Code of Practice. Available at: https://assets.publishing.service.gov.uk/government/uploads/system/uploads/attachment_data/file/435512/MHA_Code_of_Practice.PDF

Mental Capacity Act 2005: Code of Practice. Available at: https://assets.publishing.service.gov.uk/government/uploads/system/uploads/attachment_data/file/921428/Mental-capacity-act-code-of-practice.pdf

National Institute for Health and Care Excellence (NICE). 2014. SC1 Managing medicines in care homes. Available at: www.nice.org.uk/guidance/sc1

Chapter 4   Medicine formulation, routes of administration, and dosing

Chapter aims

By the end of this chapter you should be able to:

1. Explore the various routes of medicine administration and their associated advantages and disadvantages.
2. Consider how patient factors influence the way in which medicines are administered.
3. Consider the safe disposal of medicines following administration.

Introduction

Medicines are the most used interventions in healthcare. However, for any medicine to have an effect, it must first be administered to the body. There are many ways or routes to administer medicines, each associated with advantages and disadvantages. Some routes allow the medicine to be absorbed and distributed to the entire body, whilst others are designed for the medicine to have a local effect at the site of administration. This chapter will explore some of the different routes of administration, including the types of medicinal products given via different routes, and the rationale behind them.

The oral route of administration

Case study

William is a 43-year-old man with Down's syndrome and epilepsy. His father passed away several years ago, and he lives at home with his elderly mother. William is prescribed carbamazepine and sodium valproate for the management of his epilepsy. His current prescription is presented in Figure 4.1.

Name:	William Hughes		DOB: 23/9/1978	
Condition(s):	Down's Syndrome; Epilepsy			
Medicine	Formulation/route	Dose	Frequency	
Carbamazepine	Tablet	200mg	Four times a day	
Sodium valproate	E/C Tablet	500mg	Twice a day	

Figure 4.1 William's medicines

William's mother normally helps him to take his tablets, but recently she has become more confused. As a result, William has missed some doses, and suffered a seizure.

Activity 4.1 Critical thinking

Using the British National Formulary (BNF) see if you can find a way in which the dose of William's carbamazepine and sodium valproate could be given in a simpler way, with fewer doses to remember. You might need to look in the 'Indications and Dose' and 'Medicinal Forms' sections for each medicine.

An outline answer is given at the end of this chapter.

The oral route (placing a medicine in the mouth and swallowing it) is the most common way of administering medicines. It is easily accessible and convenient for the patient, and does not necessarily require the input of a healthcare professional. Once swallowed, the medicine travels through the gastrointrestinal tract, and is typically absorbed into the body, usually via the small intestine. After it has been absorbed, the drug is distributed around the body via the circulation and is able to exert its effect on a variety of body systems. Therefore, no matter which part of the body is affected by a disease, a drug given orally can often be used to treat it. In the above case study, William's epilepsy is caused by abnormal firing of nerve cells in his brain. The carbamazepine and sodium valproate he takes orally are absorbed into his body and distributed to his brain, where they help to normalise nerve cell activity and manage his symptoms.

Solid oral dose formulations

Drugs given orally are usually produced (formulated) in either solid or liquid form. William is taking two different tablets, which are examples of a solid dose formulation. Some drugs have a very unpleasant taste, and formulating them as a tablet or capsule can help to make them more palatable and more acceptable to the patient. As we have seen in previous chapters, it is important to remember that it is not only the drug that makes up the medicine formulation. The additional ingredients in tablets and capsules (for example colourings in tablets and gelatin in capsules) may need to be considered when taking a patient-centred approach to managing someone's medicines.

Modified release formulations

The length of time that a drug remains in the body after it has been taken is measured by its 'half-life'. The half-life of a drug represents the time taken for the amount of the drug in the body to reduce by half. This is an important factor to consider when deciding how many times a day a drug should be given (or dosed). Drugs with short half-lives (e.g. a few hours) need to be given several times a day in order to make sure that there is enough in the body to maintain the effect. This can be inconvenient for the patient and may be difficult to remember (as was the case with William in the case study). Drugs with longer half-lives (e.g. 24 hours) can be given just once a day, making them more convenient for the patient to take.

Most tablets and capsules start to release the drug as soon as they enter the gastrointestinal tract (termed Immediate Release or IR), which helps to enable a quick onset of the drug's effects. However, it is also possible to alter formulations so that the drug is released more slowly. This makes the absorption of the drug into the body more gradual, and in effect, extends its duration of action.

Formulations of tablets, capsules and granules that release the drug more slowly are known by a number of terms, such as controlled release, modified release, slow/sustained release and extended release. These are often abbreviated to CR, MR or SR, and XR, XL,

60

or LA, whilst branded products may incorporate an indication of the modified release property into the brand name (e.g. Epilim Chrono®). The variation in terminology can be confusing, but it is important to understand some of the differences between these formulations, as they can affect the way in which the medicine is dosed.

Many preparations with the suffix XL are dosed once a day, whilst those with the suffix MR are often dosed twice a day. However, there are exceptions, and it is important to check the BNF or the product's SmPC. Some examples of the products and their dosing are shown in Table 4.1.

Drug	Indication	Formulation	Dose frequency
Diltiazem	Hypertension/Angina	Diltiazem modified release	Three times a day
Diltiazem	Hypertension/Angina	Adizem SR® capsule	Twice a day
Diltiazem	Hypertension/Angina	Adizem XL® capsule	Once a day
Morphine	Pain	Sevredol® tablet	Every four hours
Morphine	Pain	MST® granules	Twice a day
Morphine	Pain	MXL® capsule	Once a day
Nifedipine	Hypertension/Angina	Coracten MR® capsule	Twice a day
Nifedipine	Hypertension/Angina	Adalat LA® tablet	Once a day
Quetiapine	Psychosis	Tablet	Twice a day
Quetiapine	Psychosis	Seroquel XL® tablet	Once a day

Table 4.1 Examples of drugs and their modified release formulations

Enteric coated formulations

Medicines taken orally must travel through the gastrointestinal tract before the drug is absorbed into the body. Therefore, they will be subjected to the acid conditions of the stomach. If a drug is not stable in these acid conditions, it may be destroyed before it can be absorbed, and will not have any effect. You may have noticed that William is taking an 'enteric coated' tablet. This is a tablet that has been designed to remain intact in the acid of the stomach, and only release the drug (sodium valproate) in the less acidic environment of the small intestine. A number of medicines are formulated in this way, and they allow drugs that are not stable in acid (for example the proton pump inhibitors omeprazole and lansoprazole), to be given via the oral route.

Enteric coating of tablets or capsules may also be used to try to reduce the adverse (side) effects of drugs. Some drugs may irritate and cause damage to the lining of the gastrointestinal tract. Formulating them as enteric coated preparations aims to reduce exposure of the gastrointestinal epithelium to the drug and reduce this side effect. Some non-steroidal anti-inflammatory drugs (e.g. aspirin) are formulated in this way.

We will now look at an example of how modified release tablets are managed in practice in the following case study of Catherine, as well as a related activity for you to complete.

Case study

Catherine is a 57-year-old woman with a history of bipolar affective disorder, but has suffered a stroke, and has been admitted to hospital. She takes lithium modified release (M/R) tablet (Priadel®) for the treatment of her bipolar disorder but is currently unable to swallow and has a nasogastric (NG) tube in place.

Name:	Catherine Harrison		DOB: 23/9/1964	
Condition(s):	Bipolar disorder			
Medicine	Formulation/route	Dose	Frequency	
Priadel	M/R tablet	800mg	Once a day	

Figure 4.2 Catherine's medicines

Catherine needs her lithium to prevent a relapse of her mental illness.

Activity 4.2   Critical thinking

- How could you give the lithium via the NG tube?
- Would you crush the tablet and mix it with water to pass it through the NG tube, or would you use the BNF to look for an alternative product?
- If there is an alternative product available, could you give it without first discussing with the prescriber?

An outline answer is given at the end of this chapter.

Administering modified release and enteric coated formulations

Modified release and enteric coated formulations are specifically designed to alter the way the drug passes through the gastrointestinal tract. Disrupting the formulation will affect this process, and for this reason these preparations must *not* be crushed or chewed. Crushing or chewing a modified release formulation will result in the drug being released at a faster rate than intended and may lead to adverse effects and toxicity. Crushing or chewing an enteric coated formulation will mean that the drug is no longer protected as it passes through the stomach, which may make it ineffective.

Liquid oral dose formulations

Tablets and capsules can be quite large, and swallowing them is often difficult for children and older adults in particular. This problem may be compounded by the patient tilting their head backwards when trying to swallow a tablet or capsule with a mouthful of water. It may be worth advising the patient to try tilting their head slightly downwards instead, as the solid dose will then float to the back of the mouth, making it easier to swallow. Where patients remain unable to take a solid dose form, liquid medicines are an alternative for the administration of drugs via the oral route.

Liquid formulations have the advantage of being easy to swallow (although they may have an unpleasant taste). They can typically be given via tubes such as nasogastric and percutaneous endoscopic gastrostomy (NG and PEG), although this is not always the case, so check with a senior colleague or pharmacist where necessary. The amount of drug in a liquid formulation (the strength) will usually be expressed as a weight (often in micrograms or milligrams) per volume (usually in millilitres) of vehicle (e.g. 500mg in 5mL). When working in paediatric, nursing home and care of the elderly settings you are likely to encounter a number of different liquid medicines. When administering these, it is important that you understand how to calculate the dose correctly, and that you check you have the right volume of liquid before giving it to your patient.

It is important to be aware that liquid formulations of the same drug can be available in different strengths. Once again, make sure you check the strength that you are using when calculating the amount that you need to give. Liquid medicines are often formulated so that the typical dose is given in a 5mL volume. However, this is not always the case, so care is required. Patients requiring dose adjustments such as children and the elderly may require smaller volumes of liquid. It will be necessary to measure and administer these using an appropriately sized oral syringe.

Liquid suspensions – always shake the bottle

Liquid medicines come in different formulations, including solutions (where the drug is dissolved in a liquid vehicle) and suspensions, where solid drug particles are mixed with a liquid vehicle. It is important to shake the bottle containing a liquid medicine before removing the dose and administering it to the patient. This is particularly true for suspensions, where the solid drug particles will sink to the bottom of the bottle. If the suspension is not properly shaken, the drug will remain at the bottom of the bottle, and the patient will only receive the vehicle, which will have no therapeutic effect. If this is repeated over time, and the vehicle is removed from the bottle, the drug will be suspended in a smaller and smaller volume of liquid, and therefore become more concentrated (the strength will increase). The patient will then be at risk of receiving a larger dose than intended if the bottle is subsequently properly shaken before administration.

Oral formulations – dose equivalence

Liquid and solid formulations of the same drug may not be equivalent (i.e. they may not be given in the same dose or at the same dosing frequency). Most modified release preparations are only available as tablets or capsules, so when switching from these to a liquid, it is usually necessary to give a smaller dose more frequently. In the case study of Catherine for example, Priadel® was a modified release tablet containing lithium carbonate, which is given once a day. The available liquid formulations contain lithium citrate, are not modified release, and are given twice a day. However, even some immediate release medicines do not have the same dose when given as liquids and tablets (e.g. phenytoin). You should always discuss any change in formulation with the prescriber and check the dosing regimen in the BNF or SmPC before administering the medicine.

We will now look at an example of how liquid medicines are not always used for a systemic effect in the following case study of Saeed, as well as a related activity for you to complete.

Case study

Saeed is a 51-year-old man with type 2 diabetes mellitus. He is prescribed a combination of metformin and saxagliptin to control the amount of sugar in his blood.

Name: Saeed Ali		DOB: 23/9/1970	
Condition(s): Type 2 diabetes mellitus; Constipation			
Medicine	Formulation/route	Dose	Frequency
Metformin	Tablet	500mg	Three times a day
Saxagliptin	Tablet	5mg	Once a day
Lactulose	Solution	10mL	Three times a day

Figure 4.3 Saeed's medicines

For the last two weeks, Saeed has been suffering from constipation. He mentions this to the doctor when he goes for his review. The doctor prescribes lactulose oral solution 10mL to be taken three times a day to help manage Saeed's constipation.

Activity 4.3   Research

Lactulose contains the sugars galactose and fructose chemically linked together to form a disaccharide. Do you think lactulose is safe to give to a diabetic patient like Saeed?

As this is based on your own research, there is no outline answer at the end of this chapter, however you can find further information in the text below.

Oral medicines acting on the gastrointestinal tract

In the previous sections of this chapter, we have considered medicines given via the oral route, which are absorbed into the body via the gastrointestinal tract to have a systemic effect. However, not all medicines given orally are absorbed into the body. Lactulose oral solution is an example of these. Lactulose remains in the gastrointestinal tract, and once it reaches the colon, exerts an osmotic effect. This draws water into the colon, increasing peristalsis, and softening the stool. Because the sugars that form lactulose are not significantly absorbed into the body, it is safe to give to diabetic patients such as Saeed. Another example of a medicine that acts locally in the gastrointestinal tract after being given orally is the antibiotic vancomycin. Vancomycin is given orally but is not absorbed from the gastrointestinal tract and is used in the treatment of the infection *Clostridioides difficile.*

Antacids such as aluminium and magnesium hydroxide and alginates are also intended to have a local effect despite being given orally. Most simple antacids are alkaline chemicals and exert their effect by neutralising stomach acid to relieve indigestion. However, although the site of action is the stomach, some antacid preparations also contain sodium and other electrolytes, which can be absorbed into the body. Increased levels of sodium in the body can result in increased fluid retention. This can be problematic for patients with congestive heart failure or renal impairment.

Non-oral tablet and capsule formulations

Whilst the majority of tablet and capsule formulations are designed to be swallowed via the mouth, it is important to remember that this is not always the case. Some tablets are placed under the tongue (sublingual administration). An example is glyceryl trinitrate, used to relive acute angina. Here, sublingual administration of the tablet allows rapid systemic absorption to achieve vasodilatation and relieve the symptoms of angina. Other medicines are given via the buccal cavity of the mouth. An example is the antiemetic prochlorperazine. If a patient is suffering from nausea and vomiting, this route allows convenient systemic absorption without the risk of the tablet being vomited and expelled from the gastrointestinal tract before it can be absorbed.

Some other tablets and capsules are not designed to be placed in the mouth at all. Certain inhaler devices utilise a capsule or tablet containing the drug. The formulation is placed into the inhaler device and inhaled via the airways. It is important that patients understand how to take any medicine formulation, as taking it incorrectly will reduce or even prevent it from having an effect. There are many anecdotal stories of patients swallowing capsules that were designed to be inhaled, with a resulting lack of improvement in their asthma symptoms. Just because a drug is formulated as a tablet or capsule doesn't necessarily mean that it should be swallowed. You should be aware of this and be able to explain the rationale to your patient. If in doubt check the product information before counselling your patient.

Routes for local drug administration

In the previous section, we have discussed how the oral route is convenient and commonly used for administering medicines. It is an easy and effective way of getting the drug into the blood supply, from where it will be carried to its intended site of action. As the drug is circulated around the entire body, we refer to this as 'systemic administration'.

Whilst systemic administration can be useful, it is not without disadvantages. Some drugs are not well absorbed from the gastrointestinal tract, and some undergo metabolism in the liver before reaching the circulation. This reduces their bioavailability (the amount of the administered dose that reaches the circulation). Oral systemic administration also means that larger quantities of the drug will need to be administered, so that when it is distributed through the body it will be present in sufficient concentrations to be effective at its site of action. Furthermore, because the drug is carried throughout the entire body, it may affect tissues and organs that are not its intended site of action. Both of these factors can increase the risk of side effects or adverse drug reactions.

The alternative is to administer the medicine directly to where it is needed, sometimes referred to as 'local' administration. Where this involves application to body surfaces (e.g. the eye, lung and skin) this is also known as 'topical' administration. By doing this, it may be possible for the drug to only have an effect in the area around (or local to) the site of administration, which reduces the likelihood of side effects in other parts of the body. This part of the chapter will explore some local routes of administration, and the techniques that are used when giving medicines in this way.

Activity 4.4   Research

Routes of corticosteroid administration

The drugs listed in the table below are all examples of corticosteroids that are given via different routes of administration for either local or systemic effects. Use the BNF to identify which drugs are given by which routes, and complete the table (one example has been completed for you).

Drug	Oral	Nasal	Eye	Lung	Skin	Rectal
Beclometasone						
Dexamethasone	✓		✓			
Fluticasone						
Mometasone						
Prednisolone						

Figure 4.4   Routes of corticosteroid administration

What do you think are the advantages and disadvantages of the different routes?

An outline answer is given at the end of this chapter.

In the exercise above you looked at a variety of corticosteroids that can be administered via different routes. Corticosteroids have a range of actions but are predominantly used to reduce inflammation in disorders such as rheumatoid arthritis, asthma and eczema. As with many medicines, corticosteroids have the capacity to produce notable unpleasant side effects (such as Cushing's Syndrome, fluid retention, immunosuppression, adrenal suppression and osteoporosis). Because of these side effects, it is preferable to administer these drugs 'locally' where possible, and thereby limit the systemic side effects. This may be achieved by applying the corticosteroid directly to the tissue that you wish to treat.

Local administration to the airways

Inhalation allows the local application of drugs to the surfaces of the airways and lung, and is commonly used to treat respiratory conditions such as asthma and chronic obstructive pulmonary disease. This route allows drugs to exert their effect quickly whilst minimising systemic side effects. Inhaled drugs (such as the bronchodilator salbutamol) can be administered using metered dose inhalers (MDIs), which allow the delivery of a precise amount of the drug with each activation. In more acute circumstances, drugs may be administered via the inhaled route using a nebuliser. This is a specialised delivery device in which oxygen or air is passed through a reservoir of drug to 'nebulise' it for inhalation. The drug is aerosolised in the oxygen or air, which the patient inhales over a period of minutes, allowing a large amount of drug to be delivered.

The use of MDIs can prove difficult for the patient. There are a significant number of different devices available, which in itself can cause some level of confusion for patients. The two most commonly used types require the inhalation of the drug in powder (dry powder inhalers) or aerosolised liquid (pressurised MDI) form. Powder based delivery systems may require significant respiratory effort to successfully inhale the drug (which may be an issue in patients with respiratory disease). Pressurised aerosol systems require the co-ordinated activation of the device at the same time as inhaling, which requires practice to achieve effective delivery. Whilst use of 'spacer devices' with pressurised MDIs can help to reduce the need for co-ordination, the setup and use of these requires a certain degree of manual dexterity. Patients with issues such as hemiplegia, arthritis or Parkinson's disease may find the use of spacer devices difficult or even impossible without the support of carers.

Administration technique may be the most significant factor influencing the effectiveness of inhaled medicines. It is important to check and that your patient understands how their device works, that they know how to use it, and that their administration technique is resulting in the drug being delivered effectively. Effective symptom control may also help to reduce reliever inhaler usage in patients with airways disease and contribute to the medicine's decarbonisation agenda.

Local administration to the skin

Medicine formulations designed to allow the application of a drug directly to the skin include creams, ointments, lotions and powders. Like inhalation, this route has the advantage of treating the affected area, whilst keeping systemic absorption and side effects to a minimum. In the exercise above, the creams in question contained corticosteroids, which might be applied to reduce inflammation in disorders such as eczema. However, there are a wide range of drugs that can be delivered by this route, including analgesics (such as ibuprofen gel), local anaesthetics (such as lidocaine or prilocaine cream), and antimicrobials (antibiotic, antiviral or anti-fungal creams), whilst emollients are also applied directly to relieve dry skin conditions.

Whilst the administration of formulations to the skin is relatively easy, it can be difficult to correctly judge the amount to be applied. This can result in under-dosing by patients self-administering the medicine. One way to address this is the use of the finger-tip unit (FTU), which is the amount of cream or ointment that is squeezed from a tube onto the finger between the tip and the first knuckle crease. Whilst this is still inexact and variable from patient to patient, it can be used to provide an indication of how much to apply (e.g. one FTU for each hand, or six FTUs for the chest). Another potential problem is the wet, greasy feel that can be left after application. This can be particularly problematic in ointments (which are oil based in contrast to water-based creams) and emollients, and can result in poor treatment adherence.

Local administration to the eye

Formulations such as eye-drops and eye ointments allow the direct application of a drug to the surface of the eye or the surrounding tissues (such as the conjunctiva). The corticosteroid eye-drops mentioned in the exercise above (such as dexamethasone and prednisolone) are used to reduce inflammation in conditions such as uveitis. However, eye-drops may be used to deliver a variety of different drugs. One of the more common eye-drops that you might see prescribed is chloramphenicol, an antibacterial used to treat infections. Drops to treat internal problems with the eye include the beta blocker timolol (one of a group of drugs more commonly associated with the control of hypertension) and latanoprost (a prostaglandin) both used to reduce intraocular pressure in glaucoma. Other drugs applied to the eye include those designed to dilate the pupil (such as atropine), used to facilitate ocular examination.

Formulations applied to the eye have their own drawbacks, the most obvious of which is the inability to provide a precise dose. Directions for the administration of eye-drops are typically as a number of drops rather than a precise volume or mass of the drug. When drops are applied to the eye they can be lost onto the face and are quickly removed. Eye ointments are retained in the eye for longer, and can be administered less frequently, but like those applied to the skin, they are greasy, and also cause temporary blurring of vision. For these reasons, eye ointments are often used at night.

Formulations applied to the eye must be sterile, or contain preservatives, and care must be taken when administering them to minimise the risk of infection. Other problems encountered include local irritation (which may be due to preservatives), whilst administration requires a degree of manual dexterity. As with other routes, it is important to check that your patient can use and administer the medicine effectively.

Local administration to other sites

In addition to the routes mentioned above, medicines can also be administered locally to a number of other sites to treat conditions associated with those areas. Examples include the ear, vagina and rectum. Formulations used include drops, creams and ointments, pessaries and suppositories. Whilst we might typically associate the injection of a drug with systemic effects, it is possible to inject drugs into specific areas of the body to achieve a local effect. Sometimes this involves injecting into a self-contained cavity or tissue within the body. An example is the administration of corticosteroids into arthritic joints (such as the knee) to reduce inflammation and associated pain. Whilst this is an example of local administration, it is quite invasive and presents the potential for pain and infection at the site of administration. Similarly, local anaesthetics (such as lidocaine) can be administered by subcutaneous injection to have an effect on the specific area injected.

Disadvantages of local administration – systemic absorption

Whilst the use of a local route of administration may seem an ideal solution, there are still notable problems that can be associated with this approach. When considering the local administration of corticosteroids, the most commonly encountered examples are inhaled corticosteroids (ICS), creams, and nasal sprays. Administering the drug directly to the desired tissue allows the majority of the drug's action to be focused on that tissue. However, it is important to remember that these routes are sometimes used to administer medicines for systemic effect (for example inhaled general anaesthetics). It is therefore no surprise that some of the corticosteroid administered by these routes can be absorbed into the blood supply and have a systemic effect. Another important example is the use of beta-blocker eye-drops such as timolol, which can lead to airway bronchoconstriction (particularly problematic in patients with asthma).

The level of systemic absorption can be affected by the chemical properties of the drug. This means that the systemic side effects of treatment can be reduced by careful selection of the medicine. An example of this is the corticosteroid nasal spray, used to reduce inflammation caused by hay fever. Beclometasone is widely used for this purpose (and can be bought without prescription), however, it has a systemic absorption of approximately 44 per cent. In contrast, the drug fluticasone has minimal systemic absorption and therefore a lower risk of systemic side effects.

Even if your patient is receiving a medicine designed to deliver the drug locally, you should be alert to the possibility of systemic adverse effects and observe them accordingly.

Non-oral routes for systemic administration

As noted above, the oral route is typically the preferred option when administering medicines intended to have a systemic effect. However, in some cases the oral route is not suitable, for example, the service user may be unable to take an oral medicine due to trauma or an inability to swallow safely. Furthermore, due to their physical or chemical nature, some drugs cannot be administered orally or may be better delivered by another route for patient convenience or to provide increased efficacy. This section of the chapter will explore some of the other routes by which medicines can be administered to achieve a systemic effect.

Case study

George is a 57-year-old gentleman with hypertension and type 2 diabetes. He has recently been admitted to hospital due his persistently high blood sugar, difficult to control diabetic symptoms and an episode of hyperglycaemic hyperosmolar non–ketotic coma (HONK). As a type 2 diabetic he takes oral medicines to lower his blood sugar and control his diabetes.

Name: George Browne		DOB: 5/7/1963	
Condition(s): Type 2 diabetes mellitus; High blood pressure			
Medicine	Formulation/route	Dose	Frequency
Metformin	Tablet	500mg	Three times a day
Gliclazide	Tablet	160mg	Twice a day

Figure 4.5 George's blood sugar lowering medicines (prior to admission)

On discharge, George has received a significant medication review. The endocrinology team have reduced his gliclazide and added a small dose of insulin glargine once daily, and insulin lispro at mealtimes.

Name:	George Browne		DOB: 5/7/1963	
Condition(s):	Type 2 diabetes mellitus; High blood pressure			
Medicine	Formulation/route		Dose	Frequency
Metformin	Tablet		500mg	Three times a day
Gliclazide	Tablet		80mg	Twice a day
Insulin glargine	Subcutaneous injection		6 units	Once a day in the morning
Insulin lispro	Subcutaneous injection		4 units	Inject shortly before meals

Figure 4.6   George's blood sugar lowering medicines following review

George visits the surgery where you are working. You sit in on his appointment with the practice nurse in the diabetic clinic, and George asks why he needs to use insulin. He states he is a type 2 diabetic and does not understand why he needs to use an injectable medicine. George seems concerned about still taking his oral glucose-lowering medicines and having to inject a medicine four times a day. He also does not understand why he cannot have his insulin as a tablet like his other medicines.

Activity 4.5   Reflection

Reflect upon what George has said, and how he might be feeling. Think about how you would explain the change in his medicine regime to George, and why it is important for his ongoing management.

An outline answer is given at the end of this chapter.

Unsuitability of the oral route

Although the oral route has many advantages for the administration of medicines, it does have a number of disadvantages:

- Administering drugs via the oral route will typically lead to a comparatively slow onset of action and is often not suitable for use in acute or emergency situations.
- The oral route may also be unsuitable if the drug in question causes irritation to the gastrointestinal tract or is highly unpalatable.
- Some drugs cannot be absorbed orally. Insulin and some other drugs such as adrenaline will be destroyed by digestion in the gastrointestinal tract before they can be absorbed. In the example above, George was prescribed insulin, which must be given by injection.
- After oral administration, some drugs undergo what is termed extensive first pass metabolism in the intestinal wall and in the liver. Here the drug is almost completely metabolised before it can reach the circulation, and therefore has no effect.
- The oral route is unsuitable for patients who are unable to swallow properly; for example, an unconscious patient, an uncooperative patient, or a patient who is deemed unable to swallow medication after a speech and language therapy assessment.
- The oral route is unsuitable for patients with severe vomiting or diarrhoea, which can reduce a drug's absorption.

In the circumstances above, an alternative way of delivering a drug to the systemic circulation must be found, and there are a number of options for this. The chosen route may depend upon the drug in question, and its intended use. Some commonly used examples are given below.

Administering medicines by injection

'Parenteral' is the name given to a route of delivery that does not use the gastrointestinal tract. However, parenteral is sometimes used to describe an injectable route of administration. The most commonly used injectable routes include the subcutaneous, intramuscular and intravenous routes.

Whilst administering medicines by injection has a number of advantages (discussed below), care is needed when using this route due to the use of sharps such as needles, which must be handled and disposed of safely to avoid injury and possible infection. Local irritation at the site of administration can occur, and in extreme cases can cause particularly harmful tissue damage (e.g. extravasation). Another disadvantage is that when a medicine is injected its effect cannot be easily halted if a problem occurs. Care is needed to ensure that the volume of medicine to be injected has been correctly calculated.

Intravenous injection

The intravenous route can be used to administer small volume 'bolus' injections, as well as large volume fluid infusions, along with medicines that are irritant or cytotoxic such as cancer chemotherapy, and hypertonic solutions. As the drug is administered directly into the circulation, the bioavailability is 100 per cent, meaning that none of the drug is lost to first pass metabolism, and the onset of action is rapid. Both of these factors mean that this route is useful in emergency situations, where achieving therapeutic plasma levels quickly is important.

When preparing medicines for intravenous administration, considerations needed to ensure patient safety include maintaining sterility, and observation for the presence of particulate matter and air bubbles. This is not a route that patients can typically use to self-administer medicines, strict aseptic conditions are needed, and monitoring is key to reduce the risk of extravasation.

Intramuscular injection

Intramuscular injection involves administration of a medicine into muscle tissue, typically the deltoid (upper arm), lateral thigh or gluteal muscle. In contrast to the intravenous route where solutions must be given, a number of different injection formulations (such as suspensions) can be given intramuscularly. Some of these use sophisticated formulations of the drug to achieve a long acting (sometimes referred to as a depot) effect lasting from weeks to months. Commonly used examples are contraceptives (for example, Depo-Provera®), and, in the context of mental health, antipsychotics. The use of a long-acting formulation means that the patient does not have to remember to take a tablet every day, which may be more convenient and increase medicine adherence.

Disadvantages of the intramuscular route include the need for particular injection techniques (such as z-tracking), which typically require training and practice, and are not possible by patients. Poor technique in combination with a poor understanding of anatomical markers can lead to nerve injury and damage, or administration to layers such as the dermis, rather than muscle tissue. The route can also be painful and only relatively small volumes of liquid can be administered.

Subcutaneous injection

Unlike intravenous and intramuscular injection, the subcutaneous route may allow administration by the patient. It is the typical route by which insulin is self-administered. The route offers some flexibility, as oily solutions and suspensions (such as long-acting insulin) can be administered. Disadvantages include the inability to administer irritant medicines, and absorption is somewhat slow and variable in comparison to other routes.

The transdermal route

Activity 4.6   Research

Reena is an older patient who you have been caring for, who has been taking oral morphine for pain management for an extended period. The prescriber who looks after Reena has decided to switch her from the oral morphine to a fentanyl patch.

(Continued)

73

(Continued)

Using the BNF, the electronic medicines compendium website (EMC) and resources such as the MHRA website, research the advantages and disadvantages of using the transdermal route for the administration of fentanyl.

An outline answer is given at the end of this chapter.

The transdermal route involves administration of the drug through the skin. Drugs administered in this way include fentanyl (an opioid used for pain relief), rivastigmine (used for dementia) and nicotine. The drug is typically formulated in a patch or film, which contains a reservoir of the drug that is released over a specific period (usually 24 hours or more). Once released, the drug is absorbed through the skin, and into the circulation, bypassing the liver and first pass metabolism. The patch is worn for a finite period, and then removed and replaced with a new one. The transdermal route can be used for patients who find it difficult to swallow and can be useful because the patient does not need to take a dose of medication daily.

When administering patches to patients, you avoid contact with the adhesive side (which contains the drug) to avoid inadvertent absorption. The patch should be applied to dry skin, and care must be taken to rotate the site of application to avoid irritation. This can also be a disadvantage because it is important to remember the pattern of application. The patch must also be applied to hairless skin (in order to avoid poor absorption of the drug). Patches that are damaged in any way should not be used. Patients prescribed patches should be warned to avoid heat such as saunas, and very hot baths, as these can increase absorption of the drug. When a new patch is applied, it is important to remove and dispose of the old patch correctly, as it will still contain some of the active drug.

The rectal route

Drugs administered via the rectal route are commonly formulated as suppositories. The tip (pointed end) of the suppository is sometimes lubricated with gel or water to facilitate insertion. The rectal route can be useful in unconscious patients, and for children where swallowing a tablet may be difficult. Drugs administered via the rectal route may be exposed to less first pass metabolism than via the oral route, allowing a high plasma concentration to be achieved. However, some of the vasculature of the rectum does carry absorbed drug to the liver, where metabolism can occur. The disadvantages include the fact that it is inconvenient, many adults show a degree of distaste for the rectal route, absorption is relatively slow and care must be taken not to irritate or inflame the rectal mucosa through repeated use of particular medications.

The sublingual route

The sublingual route involves administering a medicine under the tongue, usually as a tablet, but also using other formulations such as liquids and films. Typically, it results in the medicine having a quicker onset of action than the oral route. The sublingual route also bypasses first past metabolism (unlike the oral route) and as a result, more of the drug may be able to reach the systemic circulation. Like the oral route, self-administration is easily achievable by a typical patient without the intervention of a healthcare professional.

Inhalation

Whilst many drugs are given via inhalation for their local effect on the airways in the management of respiratory disease, drugs can also be given systemically via this route (for example general anaesthetics). The advantages of delivering a medicine by inhalation include a rapid onset of action, and the amount of medicine administered can be easily regulated. There are few disadvantages to the inhalation route – local irritation may cause increased airway secretion and some medicines can stimulate bronchospasm.

Non-equivalence of routes

It is particularly important to note that switching between routes may necessitate an adjustment of the dose of medicine to be administered. Just because a drug has a particular bioavailability and achieves a particular plasma concentration when administered by a particular route does not mean that an equivalent dose, plasma concentration and clinical effect will be achieved if the route of administration is changed.

Disposal of medicines after administration

Activity 4.7   Reflection

Aston is a nurse looking after a patient who is prescribed fentanyl patches for the management of pain. He wishes to dispose of a used patch that has been replaced.

What should Aston consider when disposing of the patch?

An outline answer is given at the end of this chapter.

Medicines need safe disposal in a range of circumstances. Unwanted medicines, those from deceased patients, medicines past their expiry date, and used medicines (such as patches that have been removed after use) will need to be safely disposed of according to appropriate regulations. It is important that healthcare professionals (and especially nurses) who deal with medicine administration in patients' homes, community-based care settings and hospitals understand the regulations and the reasons for their implementation. Historically, medicines would be disposed of in domestic waste, washed down the sink, flushed down lavatories, dumped illegally or given to neighbours, colleagues and friends. This is not appropriate. Medicines and administration equipment should be disposed of according to local and national policies. Many medicines, especially in community settings, may be returned to a pharmacy for safe disposal. Particular care should be taken with the disposal of controlled drugs, cytotoxic drugs and formulations such as aerosols. Irrespective of setting, care should be taken to protect the practitioner and the environment.

Chapter summary: Routes of medicine administration

In this chapter we have seen how medicines can be administered via different routes, and some of the reasons for this. Whilst the oral route is convenient and commonly used, it may not always be the most appropriate, and a number of other options are available.

To illustrate this, we can consider a patient with the respiratory illness chronic obstructive pulmonary disease (COPD). COPD is typically managed with inhaled bronchodilators and in some cases inhaled corticosteroids. This offers effective management with good tolerability. If a patient experiences a worsening of their condition, they may require an oral corticosteroid and oral antibiotics. The use of a systemic corticosteroid can have a more wide-ranging anti-inflammatory effect, and an antibiotic will treat an infection. If the patient has an infection and fails to respond to oral antibiotics, they may be treated with intravenous antibiotics, which can provide a higher plasma level, with rapid onset to treat the infection.

In the example above, the route of administration is tailored to meet the patient's needs according to the severity of illness. The ability to modify the route helps to balance therapeutic and adverse effects and to optimise patient outcome.

Activities: Brief outline answers

Activity 4.1 Critical thinking (page 59)

Both sodium valproate and carbamazepine are available as modified release tablets, which allow less frequent dosing than the immediate release alternatives. William's treatment could be reviewed by his prescriber, and amended as shown below, requiring fewer tablets, and fewer administrations each day. However, it is important to remember that medicines used for the management of epilepsy (and many other conditions) should not be changed unless by a specialist.

Name: William Hughes			DOB: 23/9/1978
Condition(s): Down's Syndrome; Epilepsy			
Medicine	Formulation/route	Dose	Frequency
Carbamazepine	M/R tablet	400mg	Twice a day
Sodium valproate	M/R tablet	1g	Once a day

Activity 4.2 Critical thinking (page 62)

Catherine's lithium could be changed from a tablet to a liquid formulation to allow it to be administered via the NG tube. However, because lithium liquid is not a modified release formulation (unlike the Priadel® tablet), the dose must be divided and given twice a day to achieve a consistent drug level in the body. Lithium liquid is also formulated as lithium citrate (rather than lithium carbonate in the tablet), so the dose is not quite equivalent. This must be taken into account when altering Catherine's prescription. It is also important to remember that some medicines may interact with the material used to make NG and other tubes, making them unsuitable to be given in this way. Therefore, decisions to change formulations and routes should only be made by the prescriber, following discussion with a pharmacist where necessary.

Activity 4.4 Research (page 66)

Drug	Oral	Nasal	Eye	Lung	Skin	Rectal
Beclometasone		✓		✓	✓	
Dexamethasone	✓		✓			
Fluticasone		✓		✓	✓	
Mometasone		✓		✓	✓	
Prednisolone	✓		✓			✓

Activity 4.5 Reflection (page 71)

George appears to feel a little confused and perhaps even upset. Explaining the rationale for the change in his medicines could help to reassure him and engage him in his treatment. The addition of insulin is part of a strategy to manage George's poor glycaemic control and reduce his risk of the complications of his diabetes. Even though he has type 2 rather than type 1 diabetes, insulin is sometimes added to the treatment regime to help improve glycaemic control.

Many medicines, including insulin, cannot be given orally. For insulin, the reason for this is two-fold; firstly, insulin is a protein and oral administration would result in digestion of the insulin in the stomach through the action of enzymes and hydrochloric acid. Secondly, insulin is a very large molecule and would not be able to easily cross the cell membranes required for absorption from the gastrointestinal tract and into the circulation. As a result, George must administer his insulin by subcutaneous injection.

Activity 4.6 Research (page 73)

One of the advantages in switching from oral morphine to transdermal fentanyl is the decrease in frequency of administration. At best, oral morphine would be taken once daily (often twice daily or more frequently if a non-SR preparation were used). The fentanyl patch would only need to be applied twice a week.

A disadvantage of the patch is lack of flexibility in dosing and dose adjustment. Small incremental doses of morphine can be easily titrated by adjusting the strength of the tablet or adding 'when required' doses of immediate release preparations such as morphine sulphate solution. The adjustment of the fentanyl dose is a little more difficult due to the nature of the patches.

Equivalent doses of fentanyl and morphine can be found in most standard medicines management texts such as the BNF, but there are several issues to bear in mind when making transitions between dosage forms. In addition to the relative potencies of the medicines and the differences in the dosage forms, there are some practical considerations. Oral medicines are familiar to patients and service users. However, understanding how to use patches, how to change them, and how they are used safely is less familiar to most service users. This is why the service user should always be at the centre of medicines management making decisions and the prescriber and wider team that support Reena need to understand how optimal pain management will be achieved if the dosage form is changed.

Activity 4.7 Reflection (page 75)

Fentanyl is a strong opioid (around 100 times more potent than morphine). A fentanyl patch may contain more than 50 per cent of the labelled amount of fentanyl even after three days of use. This is sufficient to cause serious harm or death. Patches that are not disposed of appropriately present a risk of diversion to illicit use and accidental overdose, and a number of safety incidents (including deaths) have been reported due to incorrect disposal. Discarding fentanyl patches in domestic waste or flushing them down the toilet can cause serious harm to children, pets and those who deal with waste, as well as contaminating the environment through the water supply. You should be familiar with local guidance, which typically involves folding the patch over on itself prior to disposal.

Further reading

Electronic Medicines Compendium. Available at: www.medicines.org.uk/emc#gref

A searchable repository of Summaries of Product Characteristics for medicines with Marketing Authorisation in the UK.

Lister S, Hofland J, Grafton H. (2020) *The Royal Marsden Manual of Clinical Nursing Procedures,* 10th Edition, Professional Edition. Wiley-Blackwell.

A comprehensive guide to the evidence-based practice of nursing procedures.

Chapter 5 — Adverse effects of medicines and patient safety

Chapter aims

By the end of this chapter you should be able to:

1. Describe the common types of adverse drug reaction, and how they can be managed.
2. Apply knowledge of patient factors to reduce the risk of adverse drug reactions when administering medicines.
3. Consider the risks to the nurse when managing medicines.

Introduction

Maximising safety is an essential part of medicines management and is a key focus during drug development and licensing, and, subsequently, when a medicine is used in practice in the wider patient population. To reduce the risk of harm to both patients and healthcare professionals, care is needed throughout each stage of manufacturing, prescribing, dispensing, administering (including disposing of medicines after use), and subsequent monitoring of patient outcome. A key aim is to reduce the risk of adverse drug reactions (ADRs), which can result in significant patient harm including morbidity and hospital admission and mortality.

This chapter will discuss different adverse drug reactions, as well as some of the factors that can contribute to and mitigate against them. It will also consider the risk that medicines pose to those administering and managing medicines.

Side effects, Adverse Drug Reactions (ADRs) and their classification

Case study

Asim is a 56-year-old man. Last month, Asim hurt his shoulder whilst playing cricket. He bought some paracetamol from his local pharmacy, but after taking it for two weeks, it didn't help his pain. Asim went to see his doctor, who prescribed the anti-inflammatory drug naproxen 500mg twice a day. After taking the naproxen for six days, Asim was admitted to hospital with gastrointestinal bleeding.

Due to their pharmacodynamic action and their formulation as medicines, drugs can often cause unwanted, unpleasant or harmful effects (Adverse Drug Reactions) in addition to their beneficial (therapeutic) effects. These adverse drug reactions can be relatively mild such as a headache, or severe such as an anaphylactic reaction. In the case study above, the naproxen prescribed for Asim was intended to treat his shoulder pain, but it also affected his gastrointestinal tract, leading to bleeding, possibly from a peptic ulcer. As this example demonstrates, most drugs will not only have an effect on the intended body system, but on other organs and systems as well; this phenomenon is typically referred to as a side effect. For Asim, the side effect of the drug resulted in a serious adverse drug reaction, requiring hospital admission.

It has been estimated that approximately 6 per cent of hospital admissions result from adverse drug reactions (ADRs), and with improved medicines management, many of these could be prevented (Pirmohamed et al., 2004). In addition to patient harm,

ADRs result in significant cost to health services; resources that could otherwise be used to benefit patients. Reducing the harm associated with medicines is the aim of the World Health Organisation's third global patient safety challenge: 'Medication Without Harm' (WHO, 2017). Whilst the use of most medicines is not without risk, careful consideration of the potential benefits and harms for each individual patient can help to minimise the occurrence of ADRs.

Activity 5.1   Reflection

The following patients are all experiencing adverse reactions (ADRs) to the medicines they are taking.

1. Gwen experiences tachycardia after using a salbutamol nebuliser.
2. Alison experiences an allergic anaphylactic reaction after taking penicillin.
3. Richard develops pulmonary fibrosis after taking amiodarone.
4. Ibrahim develops tardive dyskinesia associated after taking haloperidol.
5. Sian develops nausea and sweating after stopping methadone.

In each case, think about what might have caused the ADR, and how it could be managed.

As this is based on your own observation, there is no outline answer at the end of this chapter, but the text below will give you some suggestions.

An understanding of the different causes and presentations of adverse drug reactions (ADRs) can help to inform how they can be managed to minimise patient harm. ADRs can be classified in different ways. A common method is classification by 'Type', which is explained below.

Classification by Type

The 'Type' classification (known as the Rawlins–Thompson system) divides ADRs into five types labelled A–E. The medicines literature often focuses on Types A and B, whilst some systems expand upon the Rawlins–Thompson system and extend to Types F and G.

The Rawlins–Thompson system provides a way to classify ADRs and to assist with their management. It is not a perfect classification system; a deeper evaluation and analysis of the Type classification highlights overlap between some of the classifications. For example, adrenal insufficiency associated with corticosteroid therapy; this ADR could be classified as Type C (occurs after prolonged exposure to the drug), or Type E (occurring and being clinically recognised at the point of discontinuation of therapy). The next section explores the different types in more detail.

Gwen

In the first example in the boxed text, Gwen was experiencing tachycardia with salbutamol. Using the 'Type' classification, this would be a Type A or Augmented ADR. Other examples include dehydration associated with diuretics, and diarrhoea associated with antibiotics (which affect bacteria in the gastrointestinal tract). The majority of ADRs encountered in practice are Type A. These occur as a result of the pharmacodynamic effect of the drug. In addition to its effect on the airways, salbutamol can stimulate cardiac muscle, which causes the ADR tachycardia. These ADRs are dose-related, the larger the dose of salbutamol administered (or the concentration of the drug in plasma) the more likely and severe the effect. This type of ADR is most likely to occur when larger doses are prescribed or when the patient is unable to eliminate the drug (and the drug is allowed to accumulate in the body).

Type A ADRs do not usually have a high rate of mortality and can typically be managed with dose reduction or discontinuation of therapy. Where it is not possible to reduce or discontinue treatment, a lifestyle change (e.g. increase fibre in the diet to reduce constipation) may help to manage the symptoms of the ADR. In some cases, another medicine may be needed to treat the ADR of the first medicine, although this increases the risk of inappropriate polypharmacy (see later in the chapter for further information). Gwen was receiving salbutamol via a nebuliser, which delivers a relatively high dose of drug over a short period. Once the salbutamol is eliminated from the body, the tachycardia should resolve. You should carefully observe your patients for signs of Type A ADRs, and if you think a patient is experiencing one, discuss it with the prescriber or a senior colleague, as the dose of medicine may need to be reduced.

Alison

In the second example in the boxed text, Alison was experiencing anaphylaxis after taking penicillin. Using the 'Type' classification, this would be a Type B or Bizarre ADR. Other examples include Stevens Johnson syndrome associated with carbamazepine. Type B ADRs are difficult to predict from the known pharmacology of the drug. The root of these ADRs is often immunological factors; for example, many are severe allergic reactions. The adverse reaction and the patient's response are not typically proportionate to the therapeutic dose or plasma concentration.

In comparison to Type A ADRs, the mortality rate is high and the only mechanism for management is discontinuation of therapy and management of the symptoms related to the ADR. Where a history of Type B ADR is known, it is better to avoid the use of the causal medicine. Therefore, when medicines are prescribed and administered it is important to undertake a thorough patient history, and to check the allergy section of the medicine administration chart and clinical notes carefully, to identify any previous Type B ADRs. If there is evidence of these, you should seek advice before administering the medicine. Where there are signs that a patient is experiencing a Type B ADR, they are likely to need urgent medical attention.

In Activity 5.1, Alison will probably need treatment for the allergic reaction, and she should avoid penicillins in the future. However, you should also be aware that many patients who believe they have a penicillin allergy actually do not have a true allergy. This is often due to a poor recollection of a childhood experience and can lead to the avoidance of an effective treatment for infection. To address this problem, 'de-labelling' of penicillin allergy can be attempted under medical supervision. A challenge dose of penicillin is given, and the patient monitored for adverse effects.

Richard

In the third example in the boxed text, Richard was experiencing pulmonary fibrosis after taking amiodarone. Using the 'Type' classification, this would be a Type C or Chronic ADR. Another example is growth retardation in children associated with corticosteroids. Type C ADRs typically require an extended period of exposure to the drug to develop and manifest in the patient.

As these ADRs develop over time, review of the patient's dose requirement, and ongoing need for treatment is important. This should take place at regular intervals, with a view to using the lowest effective dose for the shortest duration possible to manage symptoms of the illness.

Ibrahim

In the fourth example in the boxed text, Ibrahim was experiencing tardive dyskinesia (a type of extra-pyramidal side effect of certain antipsychotics) after taking haloperidol. Using the 'Type' classification, this would usually be classified as a Type D or Delayed ADR. Another example is the appearance of neurodevelopmental disorders in the children of women who took valproate during pregnancy.

Type D ADRs are effects that do not manifest until later in drug therapy or occur at a prolonged period after exposure to the drug. Although referred to as a Type D ADR, Ibrahim's tardive dyskinesia might also be described as occurring after chronic use of haloperidol (Type C), highlighting the potential overlap between categories in the Rawlins–Thompson system.

Dose reduction or discontinuation of therapy may be possible strategies to manage these ADRs depending upon the nature of the adverse effect.

Sian

In the fifth example in the boxed text, Sian was experiencing nausea and sweating after discontinuing methadone. Using the 'Type' classification, this would be a Type E or End of Therapy ADR. Other examples include the discontinuation syndromes associated with antidepressants and benzodiazepines. Type E ADRs manifest as withdrawal reactions following discontinuation of drug therapy.

To avoid these ADRs, care is needed when discontinuing drugs associated with known withdrawal effects (such as opioids and benzodiazepines). This often involves a gradual dose reduction, sometimes over a period of months. When drugs with known withdrawal effects are initiated, you should advise patients not to stop them abruptly or without first seeking medical advice, and a plan should be in place to manage the end of treatment period.

Type F and Type G ADRs

These two subtypes of ADR are not typically included in the Rawlins–Thompson classification. However, they can be found in the wider literature. Type F ADRs describe the unexpected failure of therapy when a medicine's efficacy is reduced, resulting in an undesired clinical outcome; for example, the decreased effect of antibiotics due to resistance.

Type G ADRs refer to a drug's genotoxic effect(s) that manifest through damage to genetic material.

A tongue-in-cheek definition of Type G ADRs is also noted in the literature. The G stands for 'gaffe' or mistake, with the ADR occurring as a result of human error such as an inaccurate diagnosis, prescribing of an inappropriate drug, a dispensing error, administration error or failure to appropriately monitor response to treatment. This reminds us of the involvement of human error in the 'adverse effects' associated with medicines.

Factors increasing the risk of ADRs

Whilst ADRs can be an unavoidable consequence of using medicines, a number of external factors can increase or decrease the chance of them occurring. Human error when managing medicines, and combining medicines leading to drug interactions, can increase the risk of ADRs. The next section explores these factors in more detail.

Medicines management errors

The literature is awash with information regarding errors relating to medicines usage, which can occur in a number of different ways. A simple way of considering these errors is to categorise where they occur in the medicines management process. An awareness of the types of error that can be made may help you to detect them and avoid harm to the patient. The following section describes these errors and makes some suggestions of how to minimise their impact.

Prescribing errors

Prescribing errors occur at the initial stage of the medicines management process, where a healthcare professional makes a mistake when prescribing. Many prescribing errors are considered avoidable, but their true incidence is difficult to quantify and assess. Prescribing errors occur for a number of reasons, such as fatigue, distraction, lack of knowledge, incorrect assessment and diagnosis, and when transcribing or copying charts.

Nurses and pharmacists who support the medicines management process in dispensing, clinical pharmacy activity and safe administration are responsible for detecting and correcting prescribing errors. Examples of errors include incorrect doses, drug interactions, or contraindicated medicines being prescribed.

Dispensing errors

Dispensing errors occur at the point at which a medicine chart or prescription is dispensed for the patient. These errors can occur for similar reasons to prescribing errors such as fatigue and distraction. In the pharmacy, a failure to follow standard operating procedures (SOP), incorrect interpretation of prescribing instructions (e.g. due to poor handwriting), picking the wrong medicine, dispensing an expired medicine or mislabelling a medicine also contribute to errors. Many dispensing errors occur because of sound-alike look-alike drugs (SaLaD). These are medicines whose names sound and look the same, for example penicillin and penicillamine. Errors are compounded when the medicine packaging looks similar (or in some cases the same).

Administration errors

Administration errors occur for similar reasons to other medicines-related errors. Physical environmental factors such as distraction, fatigue and poor lighting can contribute to the wrong medicine box being selected prior to administration. Misinterpretation of prescriptions at the point of administration, dispensing and prescribing errors, poor clinical knowledge, inexperience in decision making, SaLaD and using out of date drugs all contribute to this type of error.

Drug interactions

Case studies

Richard is a 52-year-old man who experienced a deep vein thrombosis (a clot) in his leg. He takes warfarin to help reduce the risk of further blood clots. After suffering a seizure, Richard was prescribed carbamazepine (an anticonvulsant). Richard took carbamazepine for three weeks, and then experienced a recurrence of his deep vein thrombosis.

Anthony is a 67-year-old man who has atrial fibrillation. He is prescribed warfarin, an anticoagulant used to reduce the risk of blood clotting. Anthony recently twisted his ankle

(Continued)

(Continued)

whilst out walking and bought some ibuprofen from a supermarket to help with the pain. After taking the ibuprofen for three days, Anthony noticed some severe bruising on his arms and upper body.

Claire is a 52-year-old woman with heart failure and is prescribed the ACE inhibitor ramipril. Due to worsening symptoms, spironolactone was added to her treatment. After taking spironolactone for five weeks, Claire experienced tiredness and palpitations, and went to see her GP, who diagnosed hyperkalaemia (an increased amount of potassium in the body).

Tom is a 23-year-old man with an infection in his mouth. His dentist prescribes the antibacterial metronidazole. Tom arranges to meet his friend for a drink at the weekend. After drinking half of his pint of beer, Tom starts to feel nauseous and begins to vomit.

A drug interaction occurs when one drug interferes with the action of another, causing a number of different potential problems, such as;

- The effect of one of the drugs is decreased, resulting in the patient not receiving the benefit of the intended therapy.
- The effect of one of the drugs is increased, resulting in overtreatment of the patient and possible toxicity.
- A side effect can be enhanced, increasing potential harm or discomfort for the patient.
- An entirely new adverse effect is created, increasing potential harm or discomfort for the patient.

The NMC code of conduct (NMC, 2018a) states 'make sure that the care or treatment you advise on, prescribe, supply, dispense or administer for each person is compatible with any other care or treatment they are receiving, including (where possible) over-the-counter medicines'. This is an extension of the principle discussed above. Patients are complex and can have more than one thing wrong with them at a given time. It is essential that you look at the patient as whole, and not only the presenting complaint for which they are receiving treatment. You may be caring for the patient post-operatively, or in a mental health facility, but that does not mean that you can ignore their other health concerns. If the patient has multiple co-morbidities, it is possible that they will be prescribed multiple medications. This raises the possibility of drug interactions.

In the case studies above, Richard and Anthony are both taking warfarin. The dose of warfarin must be carefully titrated to ensure the patients' clotting is kept within tight limits. Too little warfarin and the patient could have a life-threatening clot, too much and the patient is at risk of dangerous bleeding. Unfortunately, warfarin can have interactions with a large number of drugs, which both increase and decrease its effect. If a patient on warfarin takes carbamazepine the action of warfarin will be decreased, and the patient will be at increased risk of clotting (as happened to Richard). Conversely, ibuprofen reduces the ability of the blood to clot, and increases the risk of bleeding (presenting as bruising in the case of Anthony). There is an additional issue related to this interaction, as ibuprofen is available to purchase from a shop without any discussion of the patient's current health status or medicines. This means that it would not appear on a patient's medicines list or GP letter if they were admitted to hospital, and may only be identified with appropriate questioning and history taking.

In the case study above, Claire is taking ramipril, an ACE inhibitor used in the treatment of heart failure and hypertension. Spironolactone is an aldosterone receptor antagonist, which may also be prescribed to treat heart failure. Both of these drugs have the side effect of causing increased potassium. If a patient takes the two drugs together, the side effect can be magnified and cause potentially dangerous hyperkalaemia.

In the case study above, Tom is taking metronidazole, an antibiotic used to fight anaerobic bacterial infections. If a patient consumes alcohol (which can be an ingredient in liquid medicines) whilst taking metronidazole, they can develop vasodilatation, increased body temperature, vomiting, blurred vision and palpitations, even though neither of these drugs would be likely to cause those effects on their own. This example also highlights how interactions can occur with food stuffs and a medicine's excipients, and not only the drug itself.

Pharmacokinetic and pharmacodynamic drug interactions

Drug interactions can be pharmacokinetic or pharmacodynamic in nature.

- A pharmacokinetic interaction occurs when one drug affects the absorption, distribution, metabolism or elimination of another drug.
- A pharmacodynamic interaction occurs when the interaction is caused by the drugs' mechanisms of action. This can be two separate drugs competing for the same binding site (e.g. on a receptor) or simply having the same effect.

In the first two examples above, two potential interactions with warfarin were discussed, one of which was pharmacokinetic and the other pharmacodynamic. When carbamazepine is given with warfarin, it induces the liver enzymes responsible for warfarin metabolism, increasing the speed at which the body can metabolise warfarin, lowering its effectiveness. This is an example of a pharmacokinetic interaction. When ibuprofen is given with warfarin, ibuprofen's anti-platelet activity combines with warfarin's anticoagulant activity to further reduce the likelihood of clotting and increase the risk of bleeding. As this interaction is due to their similar mechanism of action, it is an example of a pharmacodynamic interaction.

Identifying drug interactions

Activity 5.2   Evidence-based practice

Have a look at the drugs listed on the chart below:

Medicines to be taken regularly				Dose	
1	Date 27/5/22	Drug and form Warfarin tablet	Route Oral		breakfast
					lunch
	Prescriber's signature Dr RSY	Other directions		3mg	teatime
					night
2	Date 27/5/22	Drug and form Phenytoin capsule	Route Oral		breakfast
					lunch
	Prescriber's signature Dr RSY	Other directions			teatime
				300mg	night
3	Date 27/5/22	Drug and form Paroxetine tablet	Route Oral	20mg	breakfast
					lunch
	Prescriber's signature Dr RSY	Other directions			teatime
					night

Figure 5.1   **Drugs chart**

1. Find out what the drugs are, why they might be given, and what common adverse effects they may have.
2. Use the BNF to identify if there are any potential interactions and identify:

   a. How the interaction affects the action of the drugs involved, and the effect on the patient.
   b. How severe the interaction is likely to be.

An outline answer is given at the end of this chapter.

With so many drugs available for use, the possible number of combinations of drugs is near infinite. It is unreasonable to think that you or any other practitioner would be able to remember them all. For this reason, we have resources available to us that can assist in the checking of drug interactions. The main resource available is the BNF.

The BNF (paper version, online and app) all contain a list of known drug interactions. This allows a practitioner to check whether there is likely to be an interaction, how that interaction is likely to manifest, and how serious it might be. The BNF categorises interactions as Mild, Moderate or Severe, or unknown. Whilst all interactions should be avoided if possible, Moderate interactions are described as causing 'considerable distress' and could 'partially incapacitate' and Severe interactions may be 'life-threatening'.

Reducing the risk of ADRs

Providing medicines to a patient can be one of the most effective interventions that a healthcare professional can deliver. It is also, conversely, one of the greatest opportunities that a professional has to do harm, if a mistake is made. To help prevent errors and minimise the risk of harm all healthcare professionals involved in the administration of medications should have the appropriate level of knowledge and understanding required to do this safely (as outlined in standard 18 of the NMC Code). The following section discusses some approaches to minimise the risk of ADRs.

The 'Rs'

To support staff in the safe provision of medicines, there are various mnemonics and checklists that can help to ensure that the medicine is correct and appropriate for use. The most famous of these is the 5 Rs or 5 rights:

- Right Patient
- Right Drug
- Right Time
- Right Dose
- Right Route

These are the fundamental baseline checks that must be made by anyone involved in the administration of medicines. They are however, in themselves, insufficient to ensure complete safety, especially if they are taken at face value. Over the years many commentators have recommended extending this mnemonic to 7Rs and then 9Rs and 10Rs (Edwards and Axe, 2015) to provide a more comprehensive list of checks. Whilst these lists are all useful, no one list has been universally adopted. A useful resource, outlining what should be checked when administering medicines, is the Royal Pharmaceutical Society Professional Guidance on the administration of medicines (Royal Pharmaceutical Society, 2019).

Shortcomings of the 5 Rs

The major problem of the 5Rs is that it asks the practitioner to confirm that what is being administered matches the directions on the drug chart. It is important to consider that it is possible for a practitioner to check these five details and still cause the patient harm. This is possible because the 5Rs make two critical assumptions:

1. The drug has been prescribed correctly.

   Health care professionals with prescribing powers will have received suitable in-depth training about medicines and health conditions. As such it is reasonable to expect the medicines that have been prescribed are correct. However, human error is a feature of all processes. As such, whilst an error may be unlikely, it is dangerous to assume that it is impossible, and the nurse must be vigilant and prevent any error in prescribing reaching the patient.

2. The patient is in the same state now as when the drug was prescribed.

   The medicine may have been the perfect choice when it was prescribed, but a patient's condition can change and the choice of drug, dose, route or timing that was appropriate last week or yesterday may not be appropriate today.

Once you acknowledge how problematic these assumptions are, you can see how the 5Rs are too limited and that a practitioner must have a comprehensive knowledge of the patient and the treatment regimen in question to ensure safe administration.

The patient's condition

The NMC code of conduct states that you can only administer a medicine 'if you have enough knowledge of that person's health and are satisfied that the medicines or treatment serve that person's health needs' (NMC, 2018a). To fulfil this standard, a practitioner must therefore not only know who the patient is, but also know what *indication* (condition, disease, or symptom) the medicine is being used to treat. They must then have enough knowledge of the medicine, its mechanism of action, uses and corresponding doses to be satisfied that it is appropriate for the patient and their condition and does not interact with other treatments they are receiving (see 'drug interactions' on page 85). This knowledge is essential to truly fulfil the requirements of the 'classic 5 Rs', as the dose, route and timing of a medicine can all be influenced by the patient's condition.

There can also be situations where the drug prescribed for the patient is the correct one in principle, but other issues or co-morbidities mean that the drug is contraindicated (should not be used). An example of this might be a patient with an infection. Following cultures being sent to microbiology, it is confirmed that the bacteria causing the infection is most sensitive to amoxicillin (a penicillin), and that would be the most efficacious treatment. However, if the patient is allergic to penicillin, this is not only ill-advised, but also potentially fatal. The practitioner must have a good understanding of not only the disease being treated, but the patient's wider health status.

The nurse must also consider the status of a patient to ensure that the drug still serves their health needs. A drug may have been prescribed some time ago, but may no longer be needed, or the patient's condition may have deteriorated in such a way that the drug is no longer safe to give and is therefore 'contraindicated'. Examples might be a patient who was correctly prescribed antihypertensives due to high blood pressure, but now has dangerously low blood pressure, or a diabetic patient whose nausea and vomiting mean that they have not been eating, so their standard treatments could precipitate dangerous hypoglycaemia. Because of this, it is essential that up-to-date patient vital signs (BP, Pulse, Respiration, Temperature, Blood glucose, etc.) have been recorded before a patient is administered their medicine (in a ward environment vital signs sometimes referred to as observations or 'obs' are often completed before the drug round begins). If in doubt discuss with a senior colleague.

Medicines reconciliation and transition of care

The movement or transition of a patient from one care setting to another (such as from a residential setting to a hospital), typically involves a change in care team, a change in the method of record keeping, and often a change in the treatment regime. All of these factors can contribute to the increased risk of medicine errors, which is commonly associated with the transition of care process. Improving safety and reducing the largely preventable harm associated with this aspect of care forms part of the WHO Medication Without Harm initiative (WHO, 2019).

To reduce the risk of errors during the transition of care from one setting to another, effective medicines reconciliation is required. Medicines reconciliation involves the identification and recording of information regarding a patient's medicines. This requires good communication and a robust process to ensure that a complete and accurate record of a patient's medicine history is available to the relevant care team. If undertaking medicines reconciliation, you should identify details of prescribed medicines (including the drug and dose), 'over-the-counter' medicines purchased by the patient (including any complementary and herbal medicines), known drug allergies, and details of the patient's GP, as well as any other relevant information. An understanding of which of their medicines the patient is taking, and which of their medicines they might have chosen to stop taking, is also important. All of this information can be used to inform the appropriate treatment regime.

Polypharmacy

Polypharmacy describes the use of many medicines by a single patient, and is more prevalent in older patients with co-morbidities, who require different drugs to treat each of their illnesses. The use of multiple medicines may be necessary for such a patient, and where this is done effectively to optimise outcome using an evidence-based approach, this can be considered 'appropriate polypharmacy'. However, the use of multiple medicines can lead to an increased risk of adverse effects. Each drug will be associated with its own adverse effects, and combining increasing numbers of medicines will increase the risk of drug interactions. Patients may also find it difficult to remember to take all of their medicines reducing adherence to treatment. Where a patient does not gain the anticipated benefit from their medicines (or experiences harm as a result of their medicines), this can be considered 'inappropriate polypharmacy'. In some cases, extra medicines may be prescribed to treat adverse effects associated with existing medicines, and themselves result in additional ADRs. This 'cascade' prescribing is another example of inappropriate polypharmacy.

Review and, where necessary, optimisation of a patient's medicines will help to achieve appropriate polypharmacy and improve outcome. There are a number of approaches and guidelines to assist review of medicine regimes. In the UK, the Scottish Government has produced a number of resources, including the document 'Polypharmacy Guidance Realistic Prescribing' (Scottish Government, 2018), which includes a seven-step medicine review process. Other tools to assist medicines optimisation include the STOPP-START (O'Mahony et al., 2015), and Beers Criteria (American Geriatrics Society, 2019), which focus on specific drugs to avoid in combination, or to avoid (or in some cases initiate) in certain conditions in older people. It is important to remember that optimisation of a patient's medicine regime may involve starting an additional medicine where there is evidence to support its use. Whatever the framework used, when reviewing medicines, the patient should remain at the centre of the process, and the resulting treatment regime should deliver outcomes that are important to them.

Ongoing monitoring and review of medicines

There are a number of approaches to monitoring medicines usage in practice. These range from the monitoring and review of an individual patient, to monitoring the use of a medicine on a national or international basis. All patients treated with medicines should be reviewed to identify whether the treatment is delivering its intended benefit. In addition, a number of medicines are associated with a high risk of harm, and patients treated with these must be monitored accordingly. However, in order to identify certain adverse effects (for example those that occur less commonly), the wider usage of drugs in practice must be monitored (termed pharmacovigilance). The monitoring of individual patients, and pharmacovigilance, are discussed below.

The appropriate and safe use of medicines centres on a balance between the clinical benefit and the risk posed to the patient. Patients should be reviewed at regular intervals to ensure that they are not suffering from any adverse effects. This may involve a discussion with the patient to explore their views of the treatment and any unwanted effects. Patients may not always be confident to discuss adverse effects (for example sexual dysfunction), but these are important to explore, as they can contribute to treatment non-adherence.

Where a drug can affect the functioning of a specific organ or other tissue, monitoring may take the form of investigations such as thyroid, renal or liver function tests. These help to ensure that the relevant organ is working correctly, and will typically be specified in the Summary of Product Characteristics. In some cases, the required tests are mandated by the regulator (the Medicines and Healthcare Products Regulatory Agency in the UK), and patients cannot be treated unless the monitoring is undertaken and recorded. An example is the antipsychotic clozapine, which requires regular full blood count monitoring to manage the risk of agranulocytosis and other blood disorders. Other examples are pregnancy prevention programmes associated with lenalidomide and thalidomide (used for the treatment of certain types of cancer), and the anticonvulsant and mood stabiliser sodium valproate.

The pharmacokinetic properties of many drugs are altered in patients with renal impairment. Monitoring of renal function can help to guide dosing and minimise the risk of toxicity in these cases and is explored in more detail in Chapter 5.

Therapeutic drug monitoring

Case study

Ethel is an 84-year-old woman. She has an appointment with her General Practitioner, and you are present in the consultation. Ethel outlines that she is currently feeling nauseous, has vomited several times and describes abdominal pain and discomfort, with diarrhoea of recent onset. She has been feeling dizzy and lightheaded, very sluggish and feels like she is devoid of energy.

The only medicine that Ethel is taking is digoxin 125 micrograms daily. She receives a regular prescription, which she never fails to collect.

Activity 5.3   Research

What could be causing Ethel's symptoms? Review the electronic medicines compendium (EMC) entry for digoxin and establish the typical plasma concentration for therapeutic effect. In addition, explore the section on overdose and its management and consider the place of therapeutic drug monitoring when the patient is prescribed digoxin.

Digoxin Tablets BP 250 micrograms – Summary of Product Characteristics (SmPC) – (EMC) (medicines.org.uk)

An outline answer is given at the end of this chapter.

If an excessive dose of a medicine is taken (for example a deliberate or accidental overdose), the patient might exhibit signs and symptoms of toxicity (a Type A adverse drug reaction). Drug toxicity can also manifest at therapeutic doses due to the nature of biological variation amongst humans and the variety of factors that can affect pharmacokinetics and the homeostasis of human physiology. If drug toxicity is suspected, one way of confirming the hypothesis is to undertake therapeutic drug monitoring. Therapeutic drug monitoring is a tool used to measure the plasma concentration of drugs and can be particularly useful to confirm a suspicion of toxicity and provide a quantitative figure of the degree of toxicity in order to inform the most appropriate treatment. Therapeutic drug monitoring is most used when patients are treated with drugs that have a narrow therapeutic range, such as lithium, theophylline and certain antibiotics, such as gentamicin.

Monitoring treatment outcome

The way in which treatment outcome is assessed will vary with illness. In some cases, a specific measure can be used, such as glycated haemoglobin (HbA_{1C}) to measure glucose levels in diabetes, the international normalised ratio (INR) to assess clotting in patients receiving warfarin, and blood pressure in patients receiving antihypertensives. In other illnesses, a more subjective assessment of the level of symptoms may be required, such as in the management of pain or psychosis. Nevertheless, effective monitoring will help to determine whether the prescribed medicine is achieving the intended benefit, or whether dosage escalation or addition of another medicine is needed to improve response.

Effective monitoring of treatment outcome will also help to inform decisions to discontinue or reduce the dose of medicines where they are no longer required, or where symptoms have improved. Selective serotonin reuptake inhibitors and other medicines used in the management of depression are typically used for a defined period after the patient has improved and then withdrawn. Benzodiazepines (e.g. diazepam) and 'Z-drugs' (e.g. zopiclone) should only be used for short periods to treat anxiety or insomnia before being discontinued to reduce the risk of dependence. The dose of corticosteroids used in the management of asthma may be reduced (or 'stepped down') when symptom control is achieved, to minimise the risk of adverse effects. Treatment discontinuation or dose reduction is not without challenges. The return of symptoms, and possible emergence of withdrawal effects as the medicine is discontinued, both require careful assessment and management. Withdrawal effects may be present over an extended period, and a gradual discontinuation of treatment may be needed.

Adverse event reporting (pharmacovigilance)

Safety monitoring of medicines is an ongoing process, which starts during clinical trials and continues long after a drug has been approved for use. Whilst trials are rigorous and ensure a high degree of safety, they cannot account for rare adverse drug reactions, unusual contraindications, or every possible drug interaction. As such, it is the responsibility of all healthcare professionals to involve themselves in the process of pharmacovigilance – the continuous assessment and reporting of adverse drug reactions. This process allows our understanding of adverse drug reactions to grow over time and may result in changes to a drug's prescribing information, or where a significant risk is identified, the drug may be withdrawn from the market.

In the UK, monitoring is primarily undertaken through the Yellow Card reporting system, so named because of the yellow pre-printed proforma used for the reporting of suspected adverse drug reactions. However, suspected ADRs can now be reported via the Yellow Card App or the Yellow Card website (https://yellowcard.mhra.gov.uk/). Whilst the main focus of the Yellow Card is to report suspected ADRs in licensed medicines, it can also be used to report defective medicines, faulty medical devices, fake medicines or to report side effects or safety concerns related to herbal or alternative medicines and e-cigarettes.

The reporting of a suspected ADR using the Yellow Card system can be undertaken by anyone who has observed the reaction. It does not need to be the prescriber nor the person who administered the medicine. The reporting is also not restricted to healthcare professionals and can be submitted by the patient or by a carer or relative.

There is a concern that ADRs are generally under-reported and many reactions are observed but no action is taken. It is believed that this, in part, stems from not knowing what should be reported or whether a suspected ADR should be reported if it is already known. The following are some examples of when a Yellow card should be submitted for a suspected ADR:

- The ADR occurs with a drug that is newly licensed or is under observation.

  o This is indicated by the presence of a '▼' on the patient information leaflet, SmPC or next to the entry in the 'medicinal forms' section of the BNF monograph. In this instance all suspected ADRs should be reported even if they are mild, inconsequential, or well known. It is important to remember that this may apply to specific formulations of a drug rather than the drug itself. As such one form or brand may be under observation but others may not.

- The ADR is serious.

  o The definition of serious includes fatal ADRs, but also those which result in incapacitation, hospitalisation, haemorrhage or hormonal changes. This also includes any ADR which prolongs hospitalisation.

- The ADR is unknown.

  o As mentioned above, when a drug is licensed and made available it will have gone through extensive testing. However, it is unlikely that it will have been given to enough people to uncover rarer adverse drug reactions. It is for this reason that newer drugs are under observation, but as some ADRs may not manifest until they have been used for long periods, it is important to consider that even in well-established drugs it is possible to uncover new ADRs. Any new ADRs should be reported even if they seem mild or inconsequential.

Whilst these examples should help you know when to report an ADR using a Yellow Card, it is important to remember that there is more of a problem with under-reporting than over-reporting, and if in doubt it is best to report.

Medicines safety: Risk to the nurse

When we consider the use of medicines, our prime concern is the safety and wellbeing of the patient. However, it is also important to consider that the administration of medicines can present a risk to the healthcare professional administering the drug.

One of the most obvious and most discussed problems is the handling and disposal of 'sharps'. This primarily relates to needles used for the administration of medicines. As these are used to puncture the skin, they can be contaminated with pathogens inadvertently collected from the patient's body fluids. If these puncture the healthcare worker (or other people's) skin, they can act as an infection vector for some particularly nasty diseases (including hepatitis and HIV). This combination of 'sharp' and 'contaminated' means that specific policies must be in place for the safe disposal of needles used for administration. The exact policy and procedure may vary depending on your employer or place of work, but will typically involve the use of 'sharps bins'. These specialised containers provide a safe means of disposing of the 'sharp' and should be taken to, or be situated close to, the place of administration. The sharp can then be disposed of as soon as possible following the administration of the drug.

The preparation of medicines may involve sharps that are not directly involved in administration (and are therefore 'clean sharps'), but which still present a potential risk of injury. The drawing up and reconstitution of medicines such as antibiotic injections will require the use of needles that need to be disposed of safely. Many injectable drugs are stored in glass ampoules (sealed glass containers), which must be broken in order to extract the drug from within. Whilst the ampoules are designed to have a breakable 'neck' and may have a pre-weakened part indicated by a dot, it is still possible to cut your fingers when opening the ampoule. It is advisable to use an 'ampoule breaker', a small device to facilitate the safe opening of the ampoule to minimise the risk of injury.

It is also important to consider the potential risk from exposure to the medicine itself. When reconstituting and drawing up injections, or handling tablets, creams or patches, there is a risk that small quantities of the drug can be inhaled or absorbed through the skin. In most circumstances the quantity of drug absorbed is unlikely to be problematic, however there are occasions where adverse effects can arise. Antibiotics are widely used and a group of drugs that many nurses (particularly those in secondary care settings) will administer. Inadvertent exposure could be dangerous for a nurse with an allergy that causes anaphylaxis, although mild reactions including respiratory symptoms, rhinitis, and dermatitis are more common. Some drugs should not be handled by women who are, or who may become, pregnant. An example is finasteride, which is teratogenic and causes harm to the male foetus.

An alternate view of ADR classification

Earlier in this chapter, we focused on the Rawlins–Thompson 'Type' classification of ADRs. However, this is not the only way of classifying ADRs, and an alternative is

'DoTS'. The DoTS system considers adverse reactions from three dimensions, namely the **D**ose, **T**ime and **S**usceptibility dimensions.

This system has been developed to overcome the cross categorisation encountered in the Type classifications, which can oversimplify the complexity of ADRs. The method is a little more complex and some factors required for accurate utilisation of the DoTS system may be unknown to the clinician. However, it encourages a significant development of the knowledge of ADRs and the complex interplay between the factors that will influence the management of the ADRs.

Dose-related dimension

The dose-related category considers ADRs in three groups. ADRs can happen in a hyper-susceptibility phase, a side effect phase and a toxic effect phase. Hyper-susceptibility ADRs occur at sub therapeutic doses, for example, significant allergic responses to penicillin can occur even after exposure to the penicillin powder that may be present on the outside of a capsule. ADRs occur in the side effect phase when they manifest at normal dose and plasma ranges for the particular medicine involved. Examples here include constipation associated with the use of opiates and dehydration with diuretics. The third phase is the toxic effects phase; this includes ADRs associated with toxic plasma concentrations, for example, nausea and vomiting associated with digoxin and dizziness and blurred vision associated with lithium.

Time-related dimension

ADRs can be classified as time dependent or time independent.

Time dependent ADRs are divided into six categories: rapid onset, first dose onset, early onset, intermediate onset, late onset and delayed onset. As the names suggest, time-dependent ADRs are labelled in relation to the time of onset in relation to the administration of the drug and the relative time to the manifestation of the adverse drug reaction.

Time independent ADRs can occur at any time doing therapy. A patient may be stable on a therapy but factors such as an inter-current illness or diseases such as renal or hepatic impairment may affect the metabolism or excretion of a drug. This may result in a change in the plasma concentration and an adverse effect due to accumulation of the drug in the body.

Susceptibility dimension

This part of the classification recognises that the risk of ADRs varies between a range of individuals and can be affected by different factors. Susceptibility includes factors such as age, disease, drug interactions, exogenous factors, gender and genetics in considering the likelihood of encountering an adverse drug reaction and its severity.

Activity 5.4   Reflection

Rhys takes amlodipine for his hypertension. He feels lightheaded at the start of the therapy and his blood pressure falls after taking the medicine. The lightheadedness is quite unpleasant, and he has to steady himself when standing up. After a few doses the issue resolves and the drug manages Rhys' blood pressure without the adverse effect.

- Using the Type and DoTS classification systems, classify Rhys' ADR.

An outline answer is given at the end of this chapter.

Chapter summary

This chapter has considered a number of factors related to medicines safety. The adverse effects of medicines have different causes and can present in different ways. An understanding of these can help to guide their management and reduce patient harm. Similarly, an awareness of the factors that increase the risk of ADRs and those that mitigate against them can help to reduce the incidence of ADRs. However, it should not be forgotten that human error is a significant driver underlying the harm associated with medicines usage, and care is needed throughout the medicines management process if this is to be avoided.

Activities: Brief outline answers

Activity 5.2 Evidence-based practice (page 88)

Question 1:

Drug	Drug type	Indication	Examples of adverse effects
Warfarin	Anticoagulant	Prevention and treatment of thrombosis	Haemorrhage
Phenytoin	Anticonvulsant	Prevention of seizures	Agranulocytosis, confusion, dizziness, skin reactions
Paroxetine	Antidepressant	Depression, anxiety, obsessive compulsive disorder	Constipation, dry mouth, nausea, sexual dysfunction

Question 2:

Drug	Second drug	Effect	Severity
Warfarin	Phenytoin	Reduced effect of warfarin, and increased risk of clotting	Moderate
	Paroxetine	Increased risk of bleeding	Severe
Phenytoin	Paroxetine	Reduced effect of paroxetine with potential treatment failure	Moderate

Activity 5.3 Research (page 93)

Ethel is presenting with all of the classical symptoms of acute digoxin toxicity and this should be investigated urgently. Measuring the amount of digoxin in Ethel's blood will help to confirm this. The risk of toxicity typically increases as the plasma concentration of digoxin increases above 1.5 micrograms per litre.

There could be many reasons why Ethel has experienced digoxin toxicity; some examples include:

1. She may have taken too much digoxin deliberately or accidentally.

2. Her renal function may have declined and consequently her body is not excreting digoxin as efficiently as before.

3. She may have an inter-current illness that has changed her response to the digoxin or affected its excretion.

4. There may have been an error in the prescribing or dispensing of her supply of digoxin resulting in her taking the wrong dose.

Activity 5.4 Reflection (page 98)

Rhys was experiencing hypotension when he started treatment with amlodipine. This ADR can be classified using the different classification systems as follows:

1. Rawlins–Thompson Types – Type A. The ADR is related to the pharmacodynamic effect and the dose of amlodipine.

2. DoTS – D – side effect phase, T – first dose/ early onset and S – this is unknown as we don't have the clinical details to make the judgement.

Further reading

The British National Formulary. Medicines Guidance. Adverse reactions to drugs.

A standard text providing information about medicines use, including indications, dosing and adverse effects.

Ferner RE. (2016) Adverse drug reactions. Medicine 44(7): 416–421

A review of the classification and causes of adverse drug reactions.

Yellow Card Scheme. Medicines and Healthcare Products Regulatory Agency. Available at: https://yellowcard.mhra.gov.uk/

The Yellow Card website provides information about adverse drug reaction reporting and allows reporting of events through an online form.

Chapter 6 Medicines management across the lifespan

Chapter aims

By the end of this chapter you should be able to:

1. Describe how age and associated factors influence the risks and benefits of medicines use.

2. Describe how you might need to adapt your approach to medicines management according to age and associated factors.
3. Apply knowledge of patient factors to reduce the risk of adverse drug reactions when administering medicines.

Introduction

This chapter explores some of the factors that need to be considered when managing medicines for patients of different ages. It is arranged by age starting before birth, moving through childhood to adults, and then to older adults. Within each age group, we have tried to include the factors that are most relevant to that group. For example, most commonly we think of renal function being reduced in older adults. However, you should be aware that most of the factors discussed can apply to all patients irrespective of their age. For example, impaired renal function will affect the management of a patient's medicines whether they are 30 years old or 80 years old. Therefore, you should consider the effects of these on your patients' medicines management whatever their age.

Pre-birth medicines management

This chapter begins with a case study, which illustrates how anticipating a patient's medicines management needs can help to avoid future complications.

Case study

Emily is an 18-year-old woman who has recently experienced a number of tonic–clonic seizures. She has been diagnosed with epilepsy and requires treatment with an anticonvulsant medicine. The usual first line treatment for tonic-clonic seizures is sodium valproate; however, her neurologist prescribes lamotrigine.

Activity 6.1   Research

Use the BNF and the information available on the Medicines and Healthcare Products Regulatory Agency website (www.gov.uk/guidance/valproate-use-by-women-and-girls) to find out why Emily wasn't prescribed the usual first-line treatment for her epilepsy.

As this activity is based on your own research, no outline answer is given at the end of this chapter. However, the text below discusses some of the issues highlighted by this case.

The use of a medicine for any patient requires weighing the probable benefit against the possible risk. For women who are pregnant, or might become pregnant, a further consideration is the potential benefit or risk to the unborn child. Perhaps the best way to address this aspect of medicines management is to take account of any possible future plan to become pregnant, when initiating treatment. In the case of Emily in the case study above, she was prescribed lamotrigine as an alternative to sodium valproate for the management of her epilepsy. Sodium valproate has been associated with foetal malformations and developmental disorders in the newborn. Although it is typically a first-line choice for the management of certain forms of epilepsy, it should not be used for patients who are pregnant, or those who may become pregnant (unless they have signed up to the pregnancy prevention programme). Although Emily may not be considering a pregnancy at the moment, avoiding the use of valproate now avoids subsequent complications (such as the need to change her treatment) if she does become pregnant in the future.

The balance of benefit and risk is not always as clear as it was with Emily and can require careful consideration. Ongoing, effective treatment of the mother's condition can be important to reduce risk to the unborn child. For example, a patient experiencing a severe psychotic episode may be at risk of harming themselves and, as a result, of harming their unborn child. Effective treatment of their psychosis with an antipsychotic could reduce the risk of self-harm, and therefore reduce the overall risk to the foetus, despite any small increase in risk of harm associated with the antipsychotic.

It is also important to note that medicine use can affect fertility. Examples of drugs associated with reduced fertility in women include antipsychotics (due to elevated prolactin levels) and chemotherapy (causing ovarian damage), whilst anabolic steroids, immunosuppressants and recreational drugs such as cocaine can affect fertility in men. The use of gender affirming hormone therapy for transgender individuals poses a particular challenge in this population. Drugs taken prior to conception may also have an effect on the foetus even if discontinued at the time of conception. For example, men who participate in clinical trials of new medicines must typically agree to use contraception for a period after completing the trial. This is to prevent any adverse effects should the medicine have delayed effects on the foetus.

Medicines management in pregnancy

Before exploring this topic in detail, we will begin with a critical thinking activity.

Activity 6.2   Critical thinking

Annette has found out that she is pregnant. She has hypertension and is taking ramipril 10mg daily.

What are the possible risks and benefits to Annette and her unborn baby of continuing or discontinuing her medicines?

As this activity is based on your own critical thinking, no outline answer is given at the end of this chapter. However, the text below discusses some of the issues raised.

Safe and effective medicines management during pregnancy is fundamentally important, and pregnant women need special consideration by the healthcare team. Whilst being able to manage medicines prior to conception may be the optimal approach, many women will become pregnant whilst already taking regular medicines. Some medicines can be safely used during pregnancy and pose little risk to the developing foetus. However, some medicines may be associated with a greater degree of risk and require a careful evaluation of the potential benefits and risks posed by their use. Other medicines should be avoided in pregnancy due to a significant risk of harm to the foetus. These include thalidomide and lenalidomide used in the treatment of certain cancers, isotretinoin used for severe acne, and, as seen in Activity 6.1, the anticonvulsant sodium valproate.

Many aspects of medicines use can be guided by a well-defined evidence base constructed from meta-analyses and randomised controlled trials. It is important to note that information about medicines management during pregnancy and post-natally is often gathered from more limited sources such as case studies. Clinicians will need to make decisions based upon this more limited data, and their own knowledge of the patient. Consideration should also be given to the wellbeing of the woman and the challenges that may be posed to the pregnancy from poorly controlled medical conditions resulting from a lack of optimised medicines use. Advice from sources such as Medicines Information Centres and the UK Teratology Information Service (www.uktis.org) and UK Drugs in Lactation Advisory Service (UKDILAS) (www.sps.nhs/uk/ukdilas) can aid the decision-making process.

Continuing medicines during pregnancy

In Activity 6.2 above, we can consider the case of Annette from two perspectives, either continuing her medicines, or discontinuing her medicines, and the associated risks and benefits to her and the developing foetus, of each approach.

Effects on the mother

In most cases, medicines present no additional risk to the woman if continued during pregnancy. Furthermore, the management of conditions such as hypertension, diabetes and epilepsy are essential to the wellbeing of the woman. From this perspective, continued management of Annette's hypertension is indicated.

It is important to note that during pregnancy significant physiological changes take place. Changes in gastrointestinal motility may affect drug absorption, changes in haemodynamic parameters may alter drug distribution, and expansion of plasma volume can increase glomerular filtration and renal excretion of drugs. Hepatic blood flow and hepatic enzyme activity is also affected by pregnancy and may affect drug metabolism. Examples of drugs that may be affected by these changes include lipid soluble anti-hypertensives such as labetalol, antidepressants such as fluoxetine, and anti-retrovirals such as ritonavir. These changes to absorption, distribution, metabolism and elimination (ADME) can result in the need for dosage adjustment in order to maintain appropriate therapeutic levels and symptom control.

Effects on the foetus

The continuation of medicines during pregnancy can have detrimental effects on the developing foetus. Drugs that are harmful during the first trimester can produce congenital malformations (or teratogenesis), with the period of greatest vulnerability usually being the third to eleventh week of pregnancy. Drugs causing these effects are sometimes referred to as teratogens or being teratogenic. During the second and third trimesters, drugs may affect foetal growth and the functional development of the foetus, in addition to exerting a pharmacological or toxicological effect.

The BNF outlines some principles for managing medicines in pregnancy. These include using the lowest effective dose, only using drugs where the benefit to the mother is greater than the risk to the foetus, and where possible avoiding all drugs during the first trimester. If medicines are used during pregnancy, established drugs with the most robust evidence base should be used in preference to newer medicines where the potential harms are less well quantified. Several drugs are clearly identified as being harmful in pregnancy and should obviously be avoided, but many drugs lie in a grey area of having an unquantifiable harm, where a clinical decision must be made.

In Annette's case, her hypertension is a chronic condition that should be treated to avoid possible harm to herself and her baby. However, ACE inhibitors such as ramipril should be avoided in pregnancy. They can negatively affect foetal and neonatal blood pressure management and have an influence on foetal and neonatal renal function. Congenital malformations have also been reported in children of women who have taken ACE inhibitors during pregnancy.

As Annette has a chronic condition that requires ongoing management, her prescriber may decide that it is necessary to switch her ramipril to an alternative anti-hypertensive. Drugs such as the adrenergic beta receptor antagonist (beta-blocker) labetolol and the calcium channel blocker nifedipine have evidence to support their use during pregnancy.

Discontinuing medicines during pregnancy

If a woman discontinues her medicines during pregnancy, there are potential risks to her health. This is especially important if the medicine is used for a chronic condition such as diabetes or hypertension, or a more enduring mental health condition such as bipolar disorder. In Annette's case, discontinuing her ramipril could result in uncontrolled hypertension, which could have a detrimental effect on her health. An added complication is that hypertension can become a feature of pregnancy, and Annette's underlying hypertension could develop into a more serious condition such as preeclampsia. As discussed above, Annette's ramipril may not be an appropriate treatment choice in pregnancy, but an alternative antihypertensive may need to be prescribed.

If medicines are discontinued during pregnancy, there can also be a risk to the developing foetus. If Annette's hypertension were untreated (due to discontinuation of her antihypertensive), it could lead to low birth weight and preterm delivery of her baby (ACOG. 2019). Similarly, if a woman has a condition such as epilepsy, then the discontinuation of medicines to prevent seizures is likely to have an adverse effect not only on the woman but also on the developing child. An uncontrolled maternal condition may also pose a risk and additional challenges at the time of delivery.

As you can see from the above, the decision to continue a patient's medicines if they are planning to become pregnant or have recently found out that they are pregnant requires careful consideration. For medicines associated with a low risk of foetal harm, the benefit will generally outweigh the risk, and they can safely be continued during pregnancy. For medicines that can adversely affect the foetus, the risk of harm to both the mother and foetus must be considered if treatment is to be discontinued and another, safer alternative is not available.

Activity 6.3   Reflection

One of your patients tells you that they have just found out that they are pregnant. They are prescribed several different medicines for different conditions.

What advice you would give them regarding their medicines?

An outline answer is given at the end of this chapter.

Post-natal medicines management – breast feeding

Case study

Whilst working on a psychiatric mother and baby unit, you are looking after a new mother, Alice, and her baby. Alice wants to breast feed her baby and asks you whether it is safe because she has been prescribed the medicines shown on the drug chart in Figure 6.2.

Activity 6.4   Research

Use the BNF, or another recognised resource such as the summary of product characteristics (SmPC), to investigate whether the medicines that Alice is taking are safe to use when breast feeding.

	Medicines to be taken regularly			Dose	
1	Date 27/5/22	Drug and form Amisulpride tablet	Route Oral	400mg	breakfast
					lunch
	Prescriber's signature	Other directions			teatime
	Dr RSY			400mg	night
2	Date 27/5/22	Drug and form Lithium M/R (Camcolit) tablet	Route Oral		breakfast
					lunch
	Prescriber's signature	Other directions			teatime
	Dr RSY			400mg	night
3	Date 27/5/22	Drug and form Paracetamol tablet	Route Oral	1g	breakfast
				1g	lunch
	Prescriber's signature	Other directions		1g	teatime
	Dr RSY			1g	night

Figure 6.2   Alice's drug chart

As this activity is based on your own research, no outline answer is given at the end of this chapter. However, the text below discusses some of the issues relevant to medicines and breast feeding.

Post-natally, probably the most important medicines management considerations are whether a drug is safe to use whilst a mother is breast feeding, and whether it can affect the infant sucking reflex. Whether a drug is safe to use in breast feeding will depend upon the amount that passes into breast milk, the amount that is subsequently absorbed by the infant, and the pharmacodynamic effect that occurs after absorption. Most small molecule drugs are able to pass into breast milk and can therefore be absorbed by the infant. If they have adverse pharmacodynamic effects on the infant, they should therefore be avoided, and bottle feeding preferred. Larger molecule drugs such as insulin and adalimumab (a monoclonal antibody used in the management of inflammatory disorders) may be less likely to pass into breast milk, and will be metabolised in the gastrointestinal tract of the infant, resulting in minimal bioavailability. They are therefore generally safe to use during breast feeding.

In Activity 6.4 above, Alice is taking amisulpride, lithium and paracetamol. The SmPC for amisulpride states that it is excreted in breast milk in significant amounts, but there is little information on the effects on the infant. As a result, the decision to continue breast feeding should be based on the risk and benefit to the infant and mother (although the BNF recommends avoiding it due to lack of available data). The BNF identifies that lithium is excreted in breast milk, with a risk of toxicity to the infant. The SmPC for Camcolit® lists breast feeding as a contra-indication and recommends bottle feeding instead. Paracetamol can generally be used whilst breast feeding, because evidence suggests that the amount excreted into breast milk is too small to be harmful. Breast feeding the infant before a drug dose is due can help to reduce exposure, as the infant will be feeding when the mother's drug level is at its lowest.

Activity 6.5   Research

In addition to the possible adverse effects of a drug on the breast feeding infant, consideration should also be given to whether a drug may affect lactation.

Use the SmPCs to identify which of the following may influence lactation:

a.   Bromocriptine
b.   Ibuprofen
c.   Lansoprazole
d.   Sertraline

An outline answer is given at the end of this chapter.

Medicines management in children

This section highlights some of the medicine management considerations relating to children. Important aspects of this include drug dosing (which is typically based upon the age or weight of the child) and administration (where swallowing solid dose formulations such as tablets and capsules may be problematic). However, dosing by weight can also apply to medicines use in adults, and, for a discussion on this topic, please refer to the section on medicines management in adults later in this chapter. For a discussion on medicine formulations including liquid medicines, please refer to Chapter 4.

Consent to treatment

Case study

You are working in A&E and Sally, a 15-year-old girl, is being treated for a dog bite. Whilst her injuries are reasonably minor, she will require antibiotics and is asking for some mild pain relief. Sally lost her phone when the dog attacked her and has been unable to contact her parents. She is there on her own. Sally is legally a minor, is she able to give consent to receive this treatment?

The text below discusses some of the issues raised.

As discussed in Chapter 3, it is a well-established principle that in order to provide a medicine (or any medical care) to a patient, you must gain their consent. For that consent to be valid it must be 'informed consent'. This means that the patient has been provided with appropriate information about the medicine and can understand the potential benefits and risks of its use. As a child lacks the knowledge and understanding required to provide 'informed consent' they are considered unable to give valid consent, and this must be obtained from the parent or responsible guardian who can make a decision on the child's behalf. Generally, this principle applies to all children who are under the age of 16. Although those below 18 years of age are considered minors in law, any consent given by those of 16 years or above shall be considered as effective as that given by someone who is 18 or over (Family Law Reform Act 1969).

Whilst it is clear that a baby or small child lacks the capacity to fully understand and consent to treatment, the standing of a 14- or 15-year-old is less clear. A case can be made that that a 15-year-old patient is capable of understanding the nature and implications of treatment and should therefore be able to consent to treatment. This case was indeed made and tested in the now famous case of *Gillick v West Norfolk and Wisbech AHA* [1985]. In this case, a mother challenged the legitimacy of medical practitioners providing contraception and abortion advice to her children without her knowledge and consent. The eventual outcome of this case was the position that once a child achieves the required intelligence and understanding of a treatment to be deemed 'competent', the requirement of parental consent is no longer necessary. As the principle is a result of this court case, it is referred to as 'Gillick Competence'.

Whilst the original case related to contraceptives, and the specific guidelines set out by the judge in this case (known as the Fraser Guidelines) relate to contraceptive advice and treatment, the principle of 'Gillick competence' can be applied to other medicines and treatments. Gillick competency allows some patients under 16 years to consent to treatment. This is based on the premise that the treatment involved is in the patient's best interests and therefore Gillick competency may be overruled if it is used to refuse necessary care.

As the application of Gillick is patient and treatment specific, it should not be assumed that it is always acceptable to administer a drug to a teenager. This means that a 14-year-old may be able to consent for one drug but not another. In the *Bell v Tavistock and Portman NHS Trust*, 2020, case, the judge ruled that it is unlikely that a patient under the age of 16 years would ever be able to consent to puberty blockers used as part of the pathway for gender reassignment, as it was doubtful they could understand the long-term ramifications of this treatment. At the time of writing, this judgement had subsequently been overturned on appeal, illustrating the legal complexity of this matter in contemporary healthcare. Caution should always be used in these matters and advice sought to clarify the situation if you are at all unsure how to proceed.

Medicines licensing

The evidence to support the use of medicines in children is typically more limited than that in adults. In part, this is due to the process of medicines licensing. The clinical trials that support the marketing authorisation (licensing) of medicines typically exclude children, and as a result experience in this group is lacking. As a result, medicines prescribed for children are often used 'off-label', which may require additional governance considerations. Doses are often extrapolated from those used in adults, which may not always reflect the dose required, and can lead to adverse drugs reactions (particularly those of Type A – augmented).

Whilst children are a typical group where evidence to support the use of a medicine may be more limited, this can also apply to other stages of life. Clinical trials of new medicines usually exclude pregnant women to avoid harm to the developing foetus, as well as older adults with multimorbidities.

Medicines management in adults

This section considers how you may need to adapt your approach to communicating with patients, and how weight, sex and genetic factors influence medicines choice and dosing.

Communication

Case study

Andrew is a 25-year-old gentleman with Down's syndrome, who has been suffering with painful constipation for about a week. Andrew has suffered with constipation in the past, which has been managed with a combination of increased fluid intake, dietary change and increased exercise. You visit Andrew and his carer at home, and they ask for advice about resolving his constipation. After assessing Andrew, you decide that a medicine is required, and lactulose is prescribed by his GP. Andrew cannot communicate verbally and is likely to have limited understanding of the medicine.

What strategies might you use to communicate with Andrew and explain what he needs to know about his medicine? How could these strategies be adapted to other situations where communication may be difficult?

Encounters like the one with Andrew are common in healthcare practice. A number of patients and service users will present with barriers to communication, which can adversely affect treatment outcome. This might include hearing impairment, limited educational attainment, and language barriers (for example when caring for patients from migrant groups). One of the criticisms levelled at healthcare professionals when managing medicines is that information is offered but the way in which it is offered is poorly considered. There can be a tendency to use jargon, acronyms and medical language that is unclear. Conversely, many service users and patients experience condescending and grossly oversimplified descriptions of conditions that they understand particularly well. Find out what the patient already knows and what they would like to know about their medicines so that you can tailor both the level and amount of information to them as an individual.

The important thing to consider in Andrew's case (and in all cases) is the ability and the limitations of the service user themselves and their support network. It is our responsibility as healthcare professionals to support the service user and identify how they communicate. Whilst Andrew may be non-verbal, he may be able to use sign language, such as Makaton, and may have good general comprehension of his activities of daily living. However, in order to support this, he may need items such as charts, signs and pictographs to communicate information about his medicines. Andrew is accompanied by his carer, so inclusion of the carer in the discussion will also be important.

When providing information about medicines, consideration of general principles of good verbal and non-verbal communication is important. For example, ensure that the consultation room is as quiet as possible, use simple language delivered at an appropriate pace, use an interpreter when necessary. Remember that some patients may rely on lip-reading or non-verbal aspects such as facial expressions, which can be challenging if wearing a face mask. Provide written information or pictures as well as, or instead of, giving a verbal explanation. Written information about medicines will often be available in a number of different languages. Consider the demographics of the population that you will be looking after and explore what tools are available to assist communication with your patients. It is also important to check that the patient understands what you have said by asking questions. As you develop skills as a healthcare professional you will realise how important the principles of clear communication are in many aspects of supporting the needs of service users. These principles can be applied to assisting all service users when communicating and especially where there may be recognised barriers to communication.

Weight

Case study

Isa, who is an inpatient on your ward, is a 54-year-old lady weighing 45kg and has undergone a minor surgical operation. After surgery she is experiencing some mild pain. To alleviate this, paracetamol has been written up on the 'as required' section of her medication chart, shown below.

Medicines to be given as required										
(Maximum dose is total dose to be given in 24 hours)						**Administration**				
1	Drug and form		Indication	Dose	Frequency	Date	30/8	30/8	30/8	
	Paracetamol tablet		Pain	0.5 – 1g	4–6 hours	Time	10.00	16.05	22.15	
	Date	Max	Route	Prescriber's signature		Dose	1g	1g	1g	
	30/8/2022	3g	Oral	Dr R. Jones		Sign	BP	RS	ID	
2	Drug and form		Indication	Dose	Frequency	Date				
						Time				
	Date	Max	Route	Prescriber's signature		Dose				
						Sign				
3	Drug and form		Indication	Dose	Frequency	Date				
						Time				
	Date	Max	Route	Prescriber's signature		Dose				
						Sign				

Figure 6.3 Isa's medicines

Isa has received three doses of paracetamol in the last 24 hours, with the last dose six hours ago. She tells you that she is still in pain and asks if she can have another dose. Are you able to give Isa another dose? What advice is given in the BNF?

The text below explores the issues raised.

The dosing regimens for medicines are designed to achieve maximum benefit for the patient with minimum risk of harm. For most medicines used in adults, a single standardised dose is given to all patients. However, this presumes that the patient being treated fits within certain 'normal' physical parameters. If the patient has non-standard physical parameters, they may require a non-standard dose. Those familiar with the management of medicines in children will be accustomed to calculating specific doses based upon the child's age or weight, whilst those who may be primarily caring for adults may be less familiar with this.

In the case study, Isa has been prescribed paracetamol, a drug which we would normally consider as having a 'standard dose'. This would typically mean that she would be allowed one more dose, as the normal dosing instructions are 1g every 4–6 hours with a maximum of 4g in a 24-hour period. However, on the medication chart it indicates that she is only permitted a maximum of 3g in 24 hours and as such cannot be given another dose for the time being.

The reason for the reduced dose is that Isa weighs only 45kg. It is logical that a smaller patient will have a smaller volume of blood and other tissue, and therefore the concentration of a drug may be significantly higher than in a larger, heavier patient (where the drug would be spread throughout the larger body). Similarly, a smaller patient may have smaller organs and therefore reduced capacity to metabolise and excrete drugs. This means that toxicity may occur at lower doses. In this case giving Isa the full dose of paracetamol could place her at risk of potentially life-threatening hepatotoxicity. Conversely, in obese patients, the standard dose of a drug may be insufficient to achieve the minimum tissue concentration for the drug to be effective. Increased body mass and corresponding blood volume and lipid rich adipose tissue can affect the distribution of drugs, and as a result, a larger dose will be needed.

Instructions relating to dosing variations can be found in the BNF monograph or the medicine's SmPC. Whilst parameters such as renal and liver function have their own sections within the monograph, information related to unusual weight characteristics may be included within the 'Cautions' section. In this case the Caution section of the paracetamol monograph states that those with body weight under 50kg should have their dose adjusted based on clinical judgement. This accounts for Isa's reduced dose of 3g in 24 hours.

Sex

Case study

Joanna is an inpatient on the urinary surgical ward where you are working. She is a 58-year-old patient who is in the hospital for a minor operation. An extract of her medication chart is shown below:

Medicines to be given regularly				Dose	
1 Date 27/3/21	Drug and form Tamsulosin M/R tablet	Route Oral		400mcg	breakfast
					lunch
Prescriber's signature Dr RSY	Other directions				teatime
					night
2 Date 27/3/22	Drug and form Paracetamol tablet	Route Oral		1g	breakfast
				1g	lunch
Prescriber's signature Dr RSY	Other directions			1g	teatime
				1g	night
3 Date 27/3/22	Drug and form Codeine tablet	Route Oral		30mg	breakfast
				30mg	lunch
Prescriber's signature Dr RSY	Other directions			30mg	teatime
				30mg	night

Figure 6.4 Joanna's drug chart

You recognise the drug tamsulosin, which facilitates micturition in patients with benign prostate hyperplasia and is therefore typically used in men.

What considerations should you take into account when administering this medicine to Joanna?

The text below explores the issues raised.

When administering medicines to a patient, it is important that you understand what they are, what they do, and what they are being used for (as discussed in Chapter 5). According to the BNF, tamsulosin is indicated for use in 'benign prostate hyperplasia', although it may be used 'off-label' (discussed in Chapter 2) to treat other conditions such as overactive bladder. However, Joanna confirms that she is taking it for benign prostate hyperplasia.

The reason for Joanna taking tamsulosin is that she is a trans woman and, whilst she was assigned male at birth, has received gender affirming therapies to become a woman. Whilst this has included surgery to alter aspects of her body associated with her biological sex, she still retains her prostate gland. This means she is at risk of prostate related conditions such as benign prostate hyperplasia and prostate cancer. This will also apply to any other retained organs, which may develop associated conditions and diseases.

Patients like Joanna may have individual needs and circumstances, which must be accounted for in the management of their care. They may require gender affirming hormone therapies that present health risks (such as oestrogen which can increase the risk of thrombosis) or take hormone blockers to prevent the manifestation of unwanted secondary sex characteristics. In all circumstances, trans men and trans women deserve the same level of care and respect that is provided to any other patient, a principle that also applies to patients with Congenital Conditions of Sex Development (CCSDs) or gender-fluid patients. This includes respecting the name and preferred pronoun choice of the patient.

The example above provides a brief consideration of some complexities that may be associated with trans patients. There are also differences in physiology that can result in different responses to drugs in male and female patients, although sex differences are often less significant than other parameters (such as body weight and genetics). Whilst most medicines will be managed in the same way irrespective of the sex of the patient, women are generally more susceptible to adverse drug reactions than men. This is partly due to pharmacokinetic aspects such as reduced metabolic capacity and reduced drug elimination, as well as greater sensitivity of certain sites of drug action resulting in a larger pharmacodynamic effect. Under-representation of women in clinical trials has also contributed to a more limited evidence base in this patient group. As a result, you should be particularly vigilant for signs of adverse effects in female patients.

Genetics

Activity 6.6   Research

Jacob is a 48-year-old man who has been admitted to your ward with recently diagnosed hypertension. You are helping one of the staff nurses with the medicines administration round, and notice that Jacob is prescribed amlodipine, a calcium channel blocker, whereas Tim, who is also 48 and has hypertension, is prescribed ramipril, an angiotensin converting enzyme (ACE) inhibitor.

Use the NICE Clinical Knowledge Summaries website (https://cks.nice.org.uk/topics/hypertension/) to try to find out why the two men might have been prescribed different medicines despite being the same age.

As this activity is based on your own research, no outline answer is given at the end of this chapter. However, the text below discusses some of the issues highlighted by this case.

The response that different people have to the same dose of the same medicine can be very different. One person may experience a good therapeutic effect, whilst another experiences intolerable adverse effects, and another experiences no effect at all. For some medicines, this variation in response can be explained by genetics. Both pharmacodynamics and pharmacokinetics can be influenced by the expression of certain genes, and, in some cases, this can help to predict treatment response, predict adverse effects and guide treatment choice.

Treatment for hypertension is typically guided by age, but also by ethnicity. First-line treatment for patients from a black African or African-Caribbean background is typically a calcium channel blocker (and, in the scenario in Activity 6.6, Jacob was prescribed amlodipine). For patients under the age of 55 and from other ethnic groups, an ACE inhibitor is typically first line, and in the scenario in Activity 6.6, Tim was prescribed ramipril. This suggests that Jacob might be from a black African or African-Caribbean background, whereas Tim might be from a different ethnic group. The reason for the different treatment approaches is that patients from a black African or African-Caribbean background typically respond less well to ACE inhibitors and are more likely to experience angioedema (an adverse effect).

The case above has illustrated one example of how ethnicity or genetics can influence medicines management. However, the therapeutic and adverse effects of many medicines, as well as their pharmacokinetics, can be influenced by these factors, and testing for genetic variation is gradually becoming part of routine clinical practice. Adopting this 'personalised medicine' approach has the potential to promote more effective use of a number of medicines. Screening tools are available to assess a person's risk of experiencing adverse effects prior to treatment initiation and have been shown to be a cost effective approach to the management of certain medicines (Plumpton et al., 2019). Similarly, a patient's therapeutic response to a medicine may also be predicted by the presence of absence of a genetic variation, and the medicine may be licensed specifically for that sub-population (e.g. ivacaftor in cystic fibrosis transmembrane conductance regulator gene mutations). This is a developing area of medicines management and is likely to gain further significance over time.

Activity 6.7 Research

The influence of genetic variation is not only seen in adults. Use the BNF and the MHRA website (www.gov.uk/drug-safety-update/) to find out how old someone must be before they can use the opioid analgesic codeine, and why this age restriction is in place.

An outline answer is given at the end of the chapter.

Medicines management in older adults

Polypharmacy

Case study

Edith is a 79-year-old woman who lives in a residential care home. She has a number of different conditions and has recently been suffering from urinary incontinence. Her doctor has prescribed oxybutynin for her incontinence, in addition to her other medicines. Over the last week, Edith has become increasingly confused and disorientated, and yesterday she fell over on her way to dinner.

Edith's medicines are listed on the chart below:

Name:	Edith John		DOB: 23/11/1942
Condition(s):	High blood pressure, insomnia, urinary incontinence, gastro-intestinal reflux disease (GORD)		

Medicine	Formulation/route	Dose	Frequency
Amitriptyline	Tablet	25mg	Twice a day
Co-codamol	Tablet	8/500mg	Once a day
Ferrous sulphate	Tablet	200mg	Three times a day
Indapamide	M/R Tablet	2.5mg	Once a day in the morning
Lansoprazole	Capsule	30mg	Once a day in the morning
Nifedipine	LA Tablet	30mg	Once a day in the morning
Nytol° (Diphenhydramine)	Tablet	25mg	Once a day at night
Oxybutinin	Tablet	2.5mg	Twice a day
Senna	Tablet	15mg	Once a day at night

Figure 6.5 Edith's medicines

Activity 6.8 Research

1. In the case study, identify what each of Edith's medicines is for, and what are some of their common adverse effects.
2. What do you think might have contributed to Edith's increasing confusion and fall?

The text below considers the issues raised, and a sample answer is also given at the end of this chapter.

As people age, it is increasingly likely that they will suffer from multiple, often long-term conditions. In order to manage multiple conditions, a number of different medicines will usually be prescribed (polypharmacy). As we have seen in the previous chapter, this can increase the risk of drug interactions, and adverse drug reactions (ADRs). Where a patient's medicines have not been carefully considered and optimised for the treatment of their condition, this can lead to 'inappropriate polypharmacy'.

Falls are a particular concern in elderly patients and can be associated with significant morbidity. Medicines that contribute to the risk of falls in the elderly include opioids, antihypertensives, and sedating drugs such as benzodiazepines and 'z-drugs' (zolpidem and zopiclone), antipsychotics and other psychotropics. As with other Type A ADRs, you should observe patients for these effects and report them to the prescriber or senior colleagues to prompt a review where appropriate.

In the case study above, oxybutynin was added to Edith's treatment. This medicine is used to treat urinary incontinence and is an antagonist of muscarinic acetylcholine receptors (it has anticholinergic effects). This can help to improve urinary symptoms but can also have effects on the central nervous system, causing dizziness and confusion. Combining multiple drugs with similar pharmacodynamic effects can increase the risk of cumulative adverse effects. Edith is also prescribed amitriptyline and Nytol® (diphenhydramine), both of which have anticholinergic effects. Adding oxybutynin to her regime increases 'anticholinergic burden' and the risk of ADRs such as dizziness and confusion, which may have contributed to her fall. It could be argued that Edith is prescribed 'inappropriate polypharmacy', as her medicines may have contributed to her fall. As she appears to be experiencing adverse effects, a review and optimisation of her treatment may be necessary to achieve 'appropriate polypharmacy'.

Whilst Edith's case study has focused on a fall event, this is not the only ADR of concern. As physiological processes become less able to maintain homeostasis as we age, the pharmacodynamic effects of medicines tend to become more pronounced. This increases susceptibility to ADRs (particularly dose-related Type A ADRs). Examples of other drugs that can cause significant adverse effects (particularly in the elderly) include, but are not limited to, non-steroidal anti-inflammatory drugs (NSAIDs), antihypertensives and anticoagulants. As a result, medicine doses for elderly patients are typically lower than those for younger adults in order to reduce the risk of Type A ADRs.

Renal and hepatic function

Activity 6.9   Research

Use the BNF or the Summary of Product Characteristics to compare the dosing requirements of the beta-blockers atenolol and metoprolol for patients with renal impairment and
hepatic impairment.

As this activity is based on your own research, no outline answer is given at the end of this
chapter. However, the text below will help to explain any differences that you might find.

In the case study of Edith, we saw how combining drugs with similar pharmacodynamic
effects can lead to ADRs, particularly in elderly patients. However, aging may also be
associated with declining renal (kidney) function. As many drugs are excreted from
the body via the kidney, any reduction in renal function can result in accumulation
of drugs excreted in this way. Accumulation of the drug leads to increased plasma levels, and an increased risk of ADRs and toxicity. This is a particular problem where the
drug is water soluble. Water soluble drugs are less likely to be metabolised in the liver
and therefore tend to be excreted in their active form. If excretion is reduced, and the
active drug accumulates, ADRs are more likely to occur than with lipid soluble drugs,
which are typically metabolised before excretion.

In Activity 6.9 above, you compared the dosing of two different beta-blockers
(medicines used in the management of angina and other cardiac conditions). For
atenolol, the dose should be reduced according to a patient's renal function, with
smaller doses needed for patients with more severe renal impairment. However, for
metoprolol, no dose adjustment is required irrespective of renal function. This is
because atenolol is a water soluble beta-blocker, and its action is terminated when
it is removed from the body via the kidney. If renal function declines, atenolol will
not be removed from the body as effectively, and its effects will be increased. In contrast, metoprolol is a lipid (fat) soluble beta-blocker, and its action is terminated by
conversion to inactive metabolites in the liver. Although excretion of the metabolites
will be reduced in renal impairment, they have little pharmacodynamic effect, and
are unlikely to lead to ADRs even if they accumulate in the body. As a result, it is less
important to adjust the dose in patients with renal impairment.

In contrast to renal impairment, the BNF does not mention any dose adjustment
for atenolol in hepatic impairment. This is because it is water soluble and does not
undergo significant hepatic metabolism. Use of metoprolol requires caution in patients
with severe hepatic impairment, but not in less severe impairment. The capacity of
the liver to metabolise drugs is significant, even when patients have some degree of
impaired hepatic function. Whilst metoprolol is metabolised in the liver, the dose does
not need to be adjusted unless liver function is significantly reduced. This may be the
case in patients who are dependent upon alcohol and have liver cirrhosis.

When considering whether the drug you are administering is at the right dose, for the right patient, it is important to consider a patient's renal and hepatic function irrespective of their age. However, as noted above, renal impairment may be more common in elderly patients, and hepatic impairment in those with certain co-morbidities such as alcohol dependence and hepatitis.

Cognition, dexterity and adherence

As patients age, a number of factors can impact on their ability to manage their medicines, including cognitive ability, dexterity and vision. Cognitive decline can lead to memory impairment and reduced executive function (affecting the planning of activities) and as a result, patients may forget to take their medicines (unintentional non-adherence). This may be compounded by the complexity of treatment regimens for patients with multimorbidity. Compliance aids (such as blister packs) are often suggested as a mechanism to overcome this problem, however, their use is not without difficulties. For example, not all medicines are stable when removed from their original packaging and transferred to a blister pack, whilst adjusting doses or treatments can lead to significant medicines wastage. Furthermore, patients with cognitive impairment may not be able to manage a blister pack any more effectively than their usual containers. Alternative approaches such as simplifying the treatment regime and providing reminders may be more appropriate. Reduced dexterity can prevent patients from opening medicine packaging such as child-proof lids and blister packs, and from using inhalers and administering eye-drops. Devices such as eye-drop dispensers and easy open caps are available.

It is important to discuss the possible impact of these factors with your patients, because if they are unable to manage their medicines effectively, they will not gain the intended benefit. If you notice deterioration in your patient's condition, it may be due to unintentional non-adherence, and addressing this could have a significant effect on their quality of life.

Chapter summary

This chapter has highlighted some patient related factors that need to be considered when managing medicines. Whilst some are specific to particular periods of life (e.g. pregnancy and breast feeding), others are applicable across the lifespan. It is important to consider these factors when both administering and prescribing medicines, as a person's genetics or renal function can have a marked effect on their response to certain medicines. Without taking these into account, you cannot be certain that you are administering the right drug, at the right dose, for the right patient, and potentially serious adverse effects may occur. Some of the factors discussed are not obvious based on a person's physical presentation, and therefore awareness and consideration of the issues is needed to ensure safe medicines use.

Activities: Brief outline answers

Activity 6.3 Reflection (page 105)

What advice about medicines would you give to a patient who has found out that she is pregnant?

If a patient has found out that they are pregnant, it can have implications for their medicines management. Some medicines may be necessary for the long-term management of chronic conditions. Discontinuation of these medicines may put the mother (and as a result the unborn baby) at risk of significant harm, and the mother may need to remain on treatment throughout the pregnancy. It may be possible to discontinue certain medicines if they are for self-limiting conditions, or where the risk to the mother from the condition is low. For certain medicines where the risk of harm to the foetus is significant, an alternate medicine may be needed. However, patients should be advised not to stop any medicines until they can discuss the risks and benefits with their prescriber.

When considering treatment for conditions during pregnancy, any risk to the foetus should be balanced against any possible harm to the mother of not treating the condition. The mother should be advised to mention that she is pregnant whenever discussing any possible new medicines with a healthcare professional (e.g. the prescriber, or pharmacist if purchasing over the counter medicines). It may be possible to manage many conditions with non-pharmacological interventions, which may be preferred during pregnancy.

Activity 6.5 Research (page 107)

Bromocriptine can inhibit lactation as it acts as an agonist of dopamine receptors in the brain, and it is sometimes used for this effect. Dopamine is a neurotransmitter and reduces prolactin released from the pituitary gland through an action on dopamine receptors. Drugs that antagonise dopamine receptors, such as metoclopramide and antipsychotics, inhibit the effect of dopamine leading to increased prolactin levels, and can cause galactorrhoea as an adverse effect.

None of the other drugs listed have an effect on lactation.

Activity 6.7 Research (page 115)

In the body, codeine is metabolised to morphine (a strong opioid analgesic), which has some serious adverse effects including respiratory depression and sedation. The conversion of codeine to morphine involves the cytochrome P450 enzyme system. The activity of certain cytochrome P450 enzyme subtypes is influenced by genetic variation. Some people have very efficient cytochrome P450 enzymes (termed ultra-rapid metabolisers), and would convert codeine to morphine more effectively, leading to higher morphine levels, and increasing the risk of serious adverse effects.

There have been cases of fatalities, where children who were ultra-rapid metabolisers have been prescribed codeine.

Because their status as ultra-rapid metabolisers would not normally be known prior to prescribing, the Medicines and Healthcare Product Regulatory Agency (MHRA) advises that codeine containing medicines only be prescribed for patients over the age of 12 years, where other analgesics have been ineffective. Furthermore, codeine is contra-indicated in anyone under the age of 18 years who has undergone tonsillectomy or adenoidectomy for obstructive sleep apnoea. Further information can be found on the MHRA website (www.gov.uk/drug-safety-update/).

Activity 6.8 Research (page 116)

1. Edith's medicines, indications and some common adverse (side) effects:

MEDICATION	Indication	Examples of common adverse effects
Amitriptyline	Neuropathic pain	Anticholinergic syndrome, drowsiness
Co-codamol	Pain	Confusion, constipation, drowsiness
Ferrous sulphate	Iron deficiency	Constipation, gastrointestinal discomfort
Indapamide	Hypertension	Hypersensitivity, constipation, dizziness
Lansoprazole	GORD	Abdominal pain, fatigue, diarrhoea, insomnia
Nifedipine	Hypertension	Abdominal pain, constipation, dizziness
Nytol®	Insomnia	Confusion, dizziness, drowsiness
Oxybutynin	Urinary incontinence	Constipation, diarrhoea, dizziness, drowsiness
Senna	Constipation	Gastrointestinal discomfort (frequency unknown)

2. What do you think might have contributed to Edith's increasing confusion and fall?

The medicine that was most recently added to Edith's treatment regime was oxybutynin, which is associated with dizziness and drowsiness, and may have contributed to the fall. Several of Edith's other medicines are associated with similar adverse effects, and a cumulative adverse effect burden may also be a factor here.

Further reading

The British National Formulary. Medicines Guidance, including prescribing in children, the elderly, pregnancy, breast feeding, and renal impairment.

A standard text providing information about medicines use, including indications, dosing and adverse effects.

Scottish Government Effective Prescribing and Therapeutics Division. Polypharmacy: Manage medicines. Available at: https://managemeds.scot.nhs.uk/. Accessed August 2021.

Provides comprehensive information relating to the management of polypharmacy.

Cheek, DJ et al. (2015) Pharmacogenomics and Implications for Nursing Practice. *J Nursing Scholarship* 47(6): 496–504.

Provides an introduction to pharmacogenomics and its relevance to practice.

Tamargo, J. et al. (2017) Gender differences in the effects of cardiovascular drugs. *Eur Heart Journal – Cardiovascular Pharmacotherapy* 3: 163–82

Discusses differences in physiology and response to drugs in male and female patients.

Chapter 7 Societal implications of medicines use

NMC Future Nurse: Standards of Proficiency for Registered Nurses

This chapter will address the following platforms and proficiencies:

Platform 2: Promoting health and preventing ill health

At the point of registration, the registered nurse will be able to:

2.4   identify and use all appropriate opportunities, making reasonable adjustments when required, to discuss the impact of smoking, substance and alcohol use, sexual behaviours, diet and exercise on mental, physical and behavioural health and wellbeing, in the context of people's individual circumstances.

2.11 promote health and prevent ill health by understanding and explaining to people the principles of pathogenesis, immunology and the evidence-base for immunisation, vaccination and herd immunity.

2.12 protect health through understanding and applying the principles of infection prevention and control, including communicable disease surveillance and antimicrobial stewardship and resistance.

Chapter aims

By the end of this chapter you should be able to:

1. Describe the role of medicines in health promotion and disease prevention.
2. Appreciate the breadth of substance misuse and its impact on health and wellbeing.
3. Demonstrate knowledge of, and strategies to reduce, antimicrobial resistance.

Introduction

The previous chapters in this book have focused broadly on how medicines are managed for individual patients. However, certain aspects of medicines usage can have a significant impact on the population and society more widely. This includes the use of medicines in health promotion and disease prevention, as well as adverse outcomes such as overprescribing and medicines misuse. This chapter explores four of the impacts that medicines use can have at a societal level, namely disease prevention, misuse, antimicrobial resistance and environmental.

Medicines as part of wider healthcare strategy

Case study

Mrs McKinley is visiting her GP surgery for an appointment with the practice nurse. Mrs McKinley has type 2 diabetes, for which she takes the drug metformin. As part of the discussion with Mrs McKinley it becomes apparent that she is still consuming a considerable quantity of biscuits daily. The practice nurse makes recommendations about reducing (or even eliminating) the biscuits from her diet as it will help to control her blood sugar and may help her to lose weight, both of which would be beneficial to her health. However, Mrs McKinley is not interested and keeps saying 'can't you just give me a stronger tablet?'

As has been discussed throughout this book, medicines can be a powerful means of improving health and correcting ill health, and as such comprise a significant proportion of healthcare interventions. This has sometimes led to the accusation that healthcare professionals focus too heavily on medicines without consideration of other potential means of improving a patient's health.

This attitude can be reflected in patients as well. Some patients have such faith in the power of medicines that they look for, or even expect that their problems can be resolved simply by taking a tablet. This view can be unhelpful as it relies on treating a problem rather than preventing it. It also ignores the fact that medicines (as powerful and useful as they are) have side effects that may cause the patient additional harm, and which may require careful management, for example in combination with other medicines.

Lifestyle interventions

In the case study above, Mrs McKinley's health could deteriorate if she cannot control her blood glucose. In type 2 diabetes reduced insulin production and insulin insensitivity result in raised blood glucose, which can cause significant damage to tissues throughout the body. To lower blood glucose a patient can either take medicines or can try to reduce their sugar intake. The problem is that sweet sugary foods and drinks taste nice, and as such it may be easier for a patient to stop eating Brussel sprouts than to reduce the intake of high glycaemic index foods. Changes to lifestyle require continued effort and change in life-long behaviours. Mrs McKinley has always had biscuits with her tea and is unwilling to change that. It is easier for her to believe that her problems can all be solved by taking another tablet.

Although there is an array of medicines available to manage diabetes, they all have their own side effects and associated risks. For example, metformin, which is considered one of the safest diabetic therapies, can cause abdominal pain, diarrhoea and in some cases lactic acidosis. Other medicines that could be added to Mrs McKinley's therapies could cause additional adverse effects. Considering the potential risk to the patient's health, and not ignoring the increased cost of additional therapies, it is best to encourage the patient to improve their diet rather than simply give more medicines.

Typically, disease management should not be a matter of either lifestyle changes or medicines, but an approach that combines both. Lifestyle changes can often be important factors in improvement alongside or even instead of pharmacological interventions and may be the first line treatment option for a number of diseases. In the case of type 2 diabetes, a low-sugar diet should be attempted first, to try to prevent the need for pharmacological intervention. If an antidiabetic medicine is prescribed, this does not provide an opportunity for the patient to eat as much sugar as they want, and they will still benefit from reduced sugar intake. Other diseases where lifestyle interventions are important include hypertension, where improved diet and increased exercise may facilitate management, and respiratory diseases (such as COPD and asthma), where smoking cessation should be a priority.

As it is well known that smoking is bad for you, and particularly problematic for people with respiratory diseases, it can be surprising to see patients with these diseases still smoking. It may even be frustrating to see a patient continue with an activity that is so clearly doing them additional harm. It is, however, important to remember that patients have the right to live their lives as they choose, which might include lifestyle choices that are unhealthy. People can use things such as smoking, alcohol or food as a stress-coping mechanism, so we must be empathetic to the difficulty that changing these behaviours presents. As healthcare professionals we must be non-judgemental but do our best to ensure that patients are fully informed of the risks their lifestyle choices present and provided with support in how to achieve these changes. This may include simple education about how to improve (such as information about more healthy diet options) or may involve cessation therapies. These are particularly useful in the example of smoking, where the lifestyle change involves overcoming a physical addiction.

Medicines for disease prevention

Whilst many medicines are used for the management of specific symptoms, they are also used to prevent future complications resulting from longer-term disease processes. In the case of diabetes, the aim is not only to control blood glucose, but to reduce the incidence of cardiovascular and other complications. Similarly, statins help to reduce cholesterol, but also aim to prevent future myocardial infarctions and cerebrovascular events. This approach aims to not only reduce the risk to the individual, but to reduce the disease burden by preventing more severe ill health developing across the wider population. This public health approach to using medicines relies upon individual patients taking preventative medicines as prescribed. This can be challenging, as if a patient is not experiencing symptoms of a disease (such as high cholesterol), but the medicine used to treat it causes adverse effects, there is little incentive to continue treatment. Explaining the longer-term benefits of taking the medicine are an important part of health promotion.

Vaccination and immunisation

As discussed above, medicines are not only given to treat a condition, but may also be used to reduce the risk of future complications. Similarly, vaccines represent another way of preventing illness rather than treating it after infection has occurred. The basic concept behind a vaccine is to allow the patient to develop immunity to a pathogen without actually being exposed to the pathogen itself. When the patient is subsequently exposed to the actual pathogen the immune system can mount a suitable response, which will either entirely protect the patient or significantly reduce the severity of the illness.

The terms immunisation and vaccination are often used interchangeably, however they do have a subtle difference in meaning. 'Immunisation' refers to the development of immunity in the patient after receiving a vaccine. A vaccine is the medicine administered to a patient to facilitate the development of immunity and 'vaccination' is the act of administering a vaccine. The term vaccine derives from the development of the smallpox vaccine by Edward Jenner in the late eighteenth century and is derived from the Latin word *vaccinus*, which means 'pertaining to a cow'.

Jenner built on the understanding that exposure to a pathogen could provide protection against future infections from that pathogen (the problem being that the first infection could be serious or even fatal). Jenner noticed that people who had been infected with cowpox, a relatively mild, infective disease, were resistant to infection from the potentially lethal smallpox. He found that as cowpox is a similar enough pathogen to smallpox, the immunity that an individual develops following cowpox infection will protect them from smallpox. Therefore, deliberately infecting people with cowpox (hence the name vaccine) would protect them from smallpox.

For over a century, vaccines have been a significant part of our healthcare strategy. From smallpox to seasonal flu, they have become a regular aspect of life, and a key strategy in the management of infectious disease. The historical use of vaccines has been instrumental in the eradication of smallpox infection, and the significant reduction in the incidence of poliomyelitis. In addition, the management of more contemporary infectious diseases, and associated complications such as cervical cancer, has been greatly influenced by vaccine use.

Numerous types of vaccine have been developed, utilising different mechanisms to prime the patient's immune system to the target pathogen. This has included the use of weaker or 'attenuated' strains of a pathogen, or the use of 'dead' pathogens, both of which will generate an immune response but will not cause harm. There has also been progress in developing vaccines for non-infective diseases, priming the immune system to attack certain types of cancer cell by recognising their distinctive surface proteins.

The importance of vaccines has come into sharp focus during the COVID-19 global pandemic, where the development and roll out of a COVID-19 vaccine was an essential feature of our global response to this crisis. In this response, some newer vaccine technologies gained notoriety. These included genetically altering a virus to express the surface proteins of the COVID-19 pathogen, thereby priming the immune system to be able to respond to the actual virus when it is encountered. Another involved using lipid nanoparticles to package mRNA coded for viral proteins. When the mRNA enters a person's cells, the cellular machinery uses this mRNA to produce viral proteins, which again prime the immune system to respond to the actual virus when it is encountered. These newer strategies have allowed us to produce vaccines for a wider variety of pathogens, but still all exploit the principle of exposing our immune system to a proxy for the actual pathogen, so that it can mount a response when an exposure occurs.

Immunisation and public health

So far, we have discussed how vaccines are an effective means of protecting an individual patient, but they are also an effective means of protecting the wider population. A pathogen will typically spread from person to person, with each infected person infecting more people who will, in turn, go on to infect others. This chain of infection can be interrupted by various actions such as social distancing and the use of Personal Protective Equipment (PPE), but also through vaccination. The vaccinated individual is not only protected from the infection, they are also significantly less likely to pass it on to others and are thereby indirectly protecting those around them.

When a significant proportion of the population is vaccinated, the ability of the pathogen to spread is greatly reduced and thereby the chance of anyone becoming infected (vaccinated or not) is reduced. This benefit, often referred to as herd immunity, is important as there are portions of society who may be unable take the vaccine for health reasons (for example, immunocompromised patients, and the very young), yet they still benefit from a reduced risk of infection. A further benefit to society is the reduced burden on health services. Preventative measures such as vaccination either prevent illness or reduce its severity, reducing the necessity for additional treatment, and even admission to hospital. During the COVID-19 pandemic the importance of this was emphasised, as the large number of COVID-19 infected patients was in danger of overwhelming the capacity of healthcare providers. However, whilst this issue was highlighted during the pandemic, the principle applies to all vaccines and all forms of preventative medicine.

Vaccine hesitancy

Case study

Tiffany St Claire is a 5-year-old child who has been admitted to hospital with measles. This is surprising because children are typically provided with a measles vaccine at the age of three. When Tiffany's mother is asked about this, she says that she has never had her daughter vaccinated as it is too dangerous. She would never expose her daughter to all the toxins found in vaccines because they can cause autism and do more harm than good.

With all of the apparent benefits of immunisation, it may be surprising that the mother in the case study above has decided not to have her daughter vaccinated against measles. Unfortunately, there is a growing trend of people declining vaccination due to fear of vaccines being dangerous. Vaccine hesitancy is not a new phenomenon and was seen in the eighteenth century when vaccines were first introduced. However, the anti-vaccine movement gained momentum in the late 1990s following the publication of a paper by Dr Andrew Wakefield, which linked the MMR (measles, mumps and rubella vaccine) to the development of autism. The resulting drop in vaccine uptake impacted upon herd immunity and contributed towards serious measles outbreaks that have occurred over the last decade.

Although Dr Wakefield's research was disproved, and the journal retracted the paper, the impact of this work was to bolster the growing movement around the world that opposes the use of vaccines. The groups are often referred to as 'anti-vaxxers'. Dr Wakefield's work is still circulated by vaccine sceptics along with other ill-informed claims about their supposed dangers. These range from claims about the toxicity of the ingredients and misunderstandings over how vaccines work, to outlandish theories about microchips and magnetising of patients.

As described above, the value of vaccination to the individual and to the population more widely is significant, however it is important to remember that vaccine hesitancy stems from a place of concern. Supporting and educating patients in a non-judgemental way to help them make informed decisions regarding their health and treatment is a key role of healthcare professionals. In the case study above, explaining the benefits and risks of vaccination, based on reliable evidence, to Tiffany's mother could support her in making more informed choices in the future.

Adverse effects of vaccines

Whilst the claims made by vaccine sceptics are often totally false, it is important that as healthcare providers we do acknowledge that, as with all medicines, there is the potential for adverse effects. These may be transient and mild (such as feeling feverish) or may be severe but very rare. The potential for adverse drug reactions to vaccines was brought to the public attention in 2021 when one of the COVID-19 vaccines was found to be associated with a risk of blood clots.

As with any therapy, considering the incidence and severity of the adverse effect must be balanced against the potential risk of catching the disease. In this instance, the incidence of clots was real but small, and whilst precautions were taken to restrict the use of this vaccine in high-risk groups, the overall benefit of the vaccine was still considered to be worthwhile. Nevertheless, the way in which the risk is perceived by individuals may be different to that at a population level. If the risk of a serious adverse effect to a vaccine is one in 2 million, approximately 30 people will experience it in a country with a population of 60 million. Although this seems a relatively small number, if you are one of the people affected, the consequences will be severe. If you also perceive that you are unlikely to catch the disease in the first place, or even if you do it will not cause significant harm, the risk of the vaccine might appear to outweigh the benefit. As noted above, as healthcare professionals, it is important to stress the role of vaccination as a way of managing disease, and the associated benefit to the population and society more widely (e.g. economic benefit and quality of life).

As with all medicines, any suspected adverse effects of vaccines should be appropriately monitored, recorded and reported using the Yellow Card system. Reporting of these cases is essential in ensuring the safety of medicines and, where necessary, can inform changes in licensing or other prescribing advice to improve patient safety.

Misuse of drugs and medicines

Drug misuse can be defined as the use of a drug or medicine that is inconsistent with legal or medical guidelines. Examples of medicines that are commonly misused include opioids (such as codeine, tramadol and morphine), which are designed to treat pain but are misused instead for their euphoric effects, and pregabalin, which is used to treat neuropathic pain but is also misused for its euphoric and calming effects. However, a number of other medicines and recreational drugs are also liable to misuse. The misuse of drugs and medicines can have negative consequences for the individual through adverse effects and even death, but can also impact health services through increased resource utilisation and society more widely through the impact of drug-seeking behaviour. You should be alert to circumstances that might indicate that a patient is misusing a drug or medicine, in order to be able to intervene and help to reduce harm.

This section will consider case studies related to the misuse of prescribed medicines and recreational drugs. It will also explore the withdrawal or discontinuation syndrome associated with certain medicines (such as the Selective Serotonin Reuptake Inhibitors [SRRIs]), which often gets confused with 'addiction'.

Misuse of medicines

Case study

Alison comes for a consultation with the nurse practitioner in the surgery in which you are currently gaining experience. Alison looks very thin (estimating her BMI by appearance suggests she is very underweight), her skin is very dry and pale, and she has some difficulties focusing on the conversation in the consultation. When she stands up to be examined, she has an obvious dizzy spell, which she attempts to shrug off when offered support. Alison is requesting laxatives (senna tablets and lactulose solution) and her focus during the consultation has centred around troublesome constipation that she is experiencing. She stated she had used laxatives purchased over the counter, but the pharmacist has suggested that further medical advice should be sought to treat the constipation. Alison is very intent and insistent on obtaining the laxatives and is in a hurry because she has a taxi waiting to take her home.

A glance at Alison's medical record in the surgery illustrates a long history of laxative prescribing by a number of different practitioners. Your colleague is somewhat concerned with Alison's appearance and demeanour and undertakes a physical examination focusing on cardiovascular, respiratory, abdominal and basic neurological observations. The consultation concludes with Alison leaving with a prescription for a small quantity of laxatives and a series of follow up appointments that include a return to the surgery, a referral to a gastroenterologist and a number of bloods being taken to establish baseline parameters.

Activity 7.1   Research

1.   What do you suspect might be wrong with Alison?
2.   Why has your colleague taken the approach that they did?

As this activity is based on your own research, no outline answer is given at the end of this chapter, however the text below explores some of the issues raised.

Alison has some of the cardinal physical, emotional and behavioural symptoms of an eating disorder. The low BMI, dry and pale skin, difficulty concentrating, and dizziness are common physical signs of an eating disorder. The previous interaction with the pharmacist suggests that they may have sold laxatives to Alison on several occasions and are now concerned that the continued purchase of such medicines is suggestive of a more serious underlying disorder.

Most over the counter treatments sold by pharmacies are intended for the management of self-limiting conditions or symptoms that have been present for a short period of time, rather than the ongoing management of more complex conditions. Whilst the medicines themselves may not be traditionally thought of as addictive, this is an illustration of the misuse of a substance that is connected to a relatively serious disorder. The insistency on obtaining the laxatives is suggestive of exerting psychological pressure on the practitioner to supply the medicine, which is another indication that misuse may be a factor.

In this case, your colleague has spotted a patient who appears to be misusing medicines. The nurse practitioner is establishing some baseline parameters before the next set of treatments proceed, but it is likely that Alison may need a referral to psychiatric services in addition to the other follow up appointments made. The misuse of laxatives is a significant issue for the service user, and a range of laxatives being misused can result in the gastrointestinal system failing to function or normal bowel habit being lost. Another consideration is the reason for the laxative misuse. This could be because of an underlying organic medical condition, but could also be as a result of a more complex psychiatric disorder (such as a body dysmorphic disorder) that will also need addressing to ensure the service user's needs are fully met.

Reducing inappropriate medicines use

Case study

Whilst working in a General Practice surgery, you observe a colleague who is assisting a patient, Simon, in withdrawing from the hypnotic drug, nitrazepam. Simon was prescribed nitrazepam 25 years ago to manage a period of insomnia, but continued to collect repeat prescriptions for the medicine without being reviewed. Simon is taking 20mg of nitrazepam every night (this is greater than the licensed dose). Guidance from the local prescribing advisor is to reduce the inappropriate prescribing of many medicines including nitrazepam.

Activity 7.2   Critical thinking

1. To which family of medicines does nitrazepam belong?
2. How might Simon have ended up taking a large dose of a medicine that was primarily designed for short term use?
3. What are some of the key drivers that support prescribers in changing prescribing practice?

As this activity is based on your own critical thinking, no outline answer is given at the end of this chapter, however the text below explores some of the issues raised.

In the case study above, Simon is prescribed nitrazepam, which belongs to the family of drugs called benzodiazepines. These can be useful in managing conditions such as insomnia and anxiety; however, they should only be used for short periods of time to reduce the risk of dependence, addiction and other adverse effects. Although hypnotic drugs are intended for short-term use, many instances occurred (and still occur) where they were initially prescribed on a short-term basis, but for a number of reasons their use has continued beyond the duration intended.

The inappropriate long-term prescribing of benzodiazepines is not normally recommended, but the nature of ill health and its management is very complex. The prescriber may have decided that the benefit of treatment for Simon outweighs any risk. However, the continued usage might be due to the prescriber failing to review the medicine appropriately, or the patient requesting ongoing supplies. This is an illustration of poor medicines management, which can be very impactful upon the wellbeing of the patient. It can be challenging to address long-term usage once established. Whilst some patients may be receptive to the idea of reducing their medicines to avoid harm, some may be more resistant, and less accepting of treatment discontinuation. It may be more effective to outline the nature of the treatment, including the likely duration prior to initiation, to ensure that the patient has realistic expectations rather than trying to change behaviour once established. Being able to communicate this information effectively is an important skill for healthcare professionals.

In more general terms this type of interaction has significant impact beyond the dependence of the individual. Prescriber's time, service user time, appointment allocation, repeat prescribing and medicines budget spend are all being misused if Simon should not be using these medicines on a long-term basis. There is a true opportunity cost to consider here, and resources are not being appropriately utilised for patient benefit.

Long-term use of a number of medicines such as benzodiazepines, gabapentinoids and opioids can be associated with significant adverse effects. Strategies at an organisational level that attempt to reverse inappropriate usage of these medicines include prescribing audit and prescribing indicators, coupled with associated educational resources. Prescribing or therapeutic indicators monitor the usage of medicines that are associated with safety or other concerns. The aim is to allow comparisons between prescribing in different organisations and encourage a reduction in inappropriate prescribing to improve patient safety. Prescribing indicators are used across the UK and there are examples available on the All Wales Medicines Strategy Group (AWMSG) and Scottish Medicines Consortium (SMC) websites that illustrate contemporary prescribing monitoring.

Drug dependence and addiction

The words dependence and addiction are often used interchangeably when discussing drug misuse, but there are important differences between the two. In medical terms, dependence specifically refers to a physical condition in which the body has adapted to the presence of a drug. If an individual with drug dependence stops taking that drug suddenly, that person will experience predictable and measurable symptoms, known as a withdrawal syndrome.

According to the National Institute on Drug Abuse (NIDA), addiction is a 'chronic, relapsing brain disease that is characterised by compulsive drug seeking and use, despite harmful consequences'. In other words, addiction is an uncontrollable or overwhelming need to use a drug, and this compulsion is long-lasting and can return unexpectedly after a period of improvement. The differences between dependence and addiction may therefore be somewhat subtle, but they are important.

Recreational drugs and harm reduction

Many legal and illegal substances are misused for recreational purposes, including opioids (such as heroin), cannabis, ecstasy, alcohol and LSD. The focus of this section is to highlight harm reduction as an approach to supporting those who misuse recreational drugs.

Case study

You attend a substance misuse clinic and observe an appointment between the pharmacist and a patient, John, who regularly injects street heroin. John has presented with what appear to be infected 'track marks'. There are clear and obvious signs of infection and inflammation along the left and right arms, and he explains that he has similar issues on his left thigh.

The pharmacist prescribes antibiotics and undertakes a full consultation with the service user, including a physical assessment and acquisition of some of John's current history. John leaves with a prescription for antibiotics and signposting advice for support. The pharmacist did not chastise John for his behaviour or pursue the line of telling John that he shouldn't be abusing street heroin.

Activity 7.3   Reflection

Reflecting on the above case study, what is important about the pharmacist's approach?

As this activity is based on your own reflection, no outline answer is given at the end of this chapter, however the text below discusses some of the issues raised.

Some members of society have a view that the harm that comes to drug misusers is primarily self-inflicted and treatment is not warranted as it is a waste of resources, which is a perspective that is sometimes perpetuated by the lay press. The case above illustrates a general approach to caring for all service users irrespective of the reason why they're using a service, and could equally apply to people who smoke, are overweight, or undertake risky sports such as rock climbing or rugby, all of which can result in harm that requires medical intervention.

When managing addiction, the principle of harm reduction can support the service user at the time of presentation and will in the longer term improve outcomes. Treating the infection early and aggressively would mean that John does not become seriously unwell and could help to prevent needless death. In addition, if more time is spent treating the condition now, as well as a reduction in harm from a human perspective, there will also be a reduction in the cost to the health service. If John's infection progresses to sepsis, the treatment will be far more complex and difficult to manage.

Harm reduction refers to policies and practices that try to reduce the harm that people do to themselves or others as a result of their drug use. It can be contrasted with primary prevention, which tries to prevent people using drugs in the first place, or to stop them using once they've started. Harm reduction first became a widely used term in the UK in the 1980s in response to the increasing number of cases of HIV among drug injectors and the development of syringe exchange schemes. Harm reduction focuses on 'safer' drug use and has also been developed as a way of educating people about drug use, rather than telling them to 'Just Say No'. The approach is illustrated on the 'FRANK' website (www.talktofrank.com), which provides information on substance use.

A clinical encounter, such as the one with John, is an opportunity to encourage the service user to interact with supporting services that are available for substance misusers in the area, and to emphasise the importance of not injecting substances. Injection can result in transmission of viruses if needles and injecting equipment are shared, and misuse of the delicate vascular system can result in other harms above and beyond those associated with the substance that is misused.

Withdrawal effects associated with medicines

Case study

Agnetha comes into the surgery for an appointment with the practice nurse to obtain a repeat prescription of her oral contraceptive. When asked how she has been feeling, she says that she has been increasingly anxious over the last two weeks, has had difficulty sleeping, and has been experiencing strange electric shock sensations in her arms. The practice nurse asks Agnetha whether she has made any changes in her life that might have caused these symptoms. Agnetha explains that she decided to stop her escitalopram just over two weeks ago, as she felt she didn't need to take it anymore.

Activity 7.4 Critical thinking

What might have caused Agnetha's symptoms, and how could other patients prevent this from happening to them?

As this activity is based on your own critical thinking, no outline answer is given at the end of this chapter, however, the text below explores some of the issues raised.

Agnetha's symptoms have probably resulted from abrupt discontinuation of her anti-depressant (escitalopram), and associated withdrawal effects (an example of a Type E adverse drug reaction). Symptoms associated with anti-depressant discontinuation vary according to the drug and its duration of use, but include restlessness, insomnia, unsteadiness, sweating, stomach problems and electric shock sensations. Some of these are similar to the common signs and symptoms associated with benzodiazepine withdrawal, which include sweating, insomnia, headache, tremor, nausea, palpitations, anxiety, depression, panic attacks and, more rarely, psychosis and seizures. Medicines such as benzodiazepines, antidepressants and beta-blockers have specific warnings advising not to abruptly stop taking them due to the associated consequences of withdrawal. This should be highlighted to the patient when the drug is initiated, to avoid problems such as those experienced by Agnetha.

It is important that patients speak to an appropriately qualified healthcare professional before discontinuing a medicine, especially those associated with withdrawal effects. There are strategies to manage planned withdrawal (e.g. gradual dose reduction and cross tapering to another medicine), whereas unplanned discontinuation can leave challenging symptoms to be diagnosed and managed. Discontinuation of antidepressants and other drugs associated with withdrawal effects should normally involve a slow reduction of the dose of the drug over a period of time before stopping. The rate of discontinuation can normally be determined from available guidelines, although it may need to be tailored to the individual patient and adjusted accordingly. Depending upon the dose and duration of treatment prior to discontinuation, this may take weeks, months or even longer. When discontinuing benzodiazepines, the original benzodiazepine is sometimes switched to an equivalent dose of diazepam, and the dose of diazepam is slowly reduced over a period of time.

The emergence of withdrawal effects may lead to the continued prescribing of a medicine to prevent symptoms occurring, despite treatment no longer being indicated to manage the original condition. This can apply to medicines that are not necessarily associated with addiction, such as proton pump inhibitors and in the example of Agnetha, antidepressants. Patients may feel powerless and unable to discontinue treatment, whilst ongoing prescribing can lead to harm due to adverse effects. Where a drug is, or has been, extensively prescribed (for example benzodiazepines), management of these adverse effects become a significant public health concern with an impact on the wider health system.

Antimicrobial resistance

Case study

Dorothy is a 58-year-old woman with no significant medical history, who works as an occupational therapist. Last year, she experienced an uncomplicated lower urinary tract infection, presenting with increased frequency and discomfort when passing urine. Her practice nurse prescribed the antibacterial drug trimethoprim to treat the infection, which resolved after three days of treatment.

Last week, Dorothy experienced another lower urinary tract infection, and was again prescribed trimethoprim by the practice nurse. On this occasion, after completing the three-day course of treatment, Dorothy's infection had still not resolved. She returned to see the practice nurse, who prescribed a different antibacterial, nitrofurantoin. After completing the course of nitrofurantoin, Dorothy's infection resolved.

Activity 7.5   Critical thinking

Why might Dorothy's second urinary tract infection not have responded to treatment with trimethoprim, when the previous infection was resolved using this drug?

As this activity is based on your own critical thinking, no outline answer is given at the end of this chapter, however the text below explores some of the issues raised.

There are a number of possible reasons for a patient's symptoms or illness failing to respond to a medicine. The diagnosis of their condition may have been incorrect, and an inappropriate medicine prescribed that is not an effective treatment for their actual condition. There may have been a prescribing or dispensing error resulting in the patient receiving the wrong medicine. The patient may have a genetic variation resulting in accelerated drug metabolism, or may be taking an interacting drug, both of which could lead to a loss of effect. The patient may not be taking their medicine or may not be taking it in the correct way. Furthermore, it should also be noted that most medicines are not effective for all patients, and only a percentage of patients will respond, even if it is taken as prescribed.

In the case of Dorothy, although the factors mentioned above cannot be excluded, the failure of her infection to resolve following treatment with trimethoprim is likely to be due to antimicrobial resistance. Antimicrobial resistance describes a situation where a micro-organism is no longer susceptible to the effects of a drug that is designed to inhibit its growth or to kill it. As a result, infections that are caused by the micro-organism will not respond to treatment with that drug and will require an alternative. Whilst we might typically think of bacterial infections in the context of antimicrobial resistance, other micro-organisms such as viruses and fungi can also exhibit this property. We therefore see resistance to antibacterial, antiviral and antifungal drugs, with similar implications for the management of any associated infection.

Causes of antimicrobial resistance

At the level of the micro-organism, resistance to antimicrobial drugs can be related to the structure of the organism, and the action of the drug. For example, if a drug is designed to interact with a specific target on or within the organism, but that target is not present or has been altered, the drug will not be effective. Alternatively, the organism may be able to inactivate the drug or prevent it from reaching its target.

The development of these mechanisms of resistance is often driven by previous exposure of the organism to the drug, which results in adaption of the organism in some way. Here, the wider prescribing and use of the drug in the general population becomes a key factor. The greater the use of a drug, the more likely it is that organisms will be exposed to it, and the more likely it is that resistance will develop. Antibacterials have also been widely used in farming as an animal food additive, contributing to their overall usage, although the precise extent of this is difficult to quantify. In the UK, trimethoprim (prescribed for Dorothy) has been extensively prescribed for the treatment of bacterial urinary tract infections, and the organisms causing them are often resistant to this drug. As a result, other antibacterial drugs such as nitrofurantoin may now be preferred as first line treatment, depending upon local resistance patterns.

In addition to the link between antibacterial resistance and higher levels of prescribing generally, the type of antibacterial prescribed is also a factor. Antibacterial drugs can be considered to have a broad or narrow spectrum of activity. Broad spectrum drugs such as co-amoxiclav, quinolones and certain cefalosporins are effective against a wide range of bacteria but are also more strongly implicated in the development of resistance. For non life-threatening infections, the use of narrow spectrum drugs such as phenoxymethylpenicillin (penicillin V) and erythromycin should normally be preferred.

Implications of antimicrobial resistance

Perhaps the most obvious implication of antimicrobial resistance is the failure of an infection to respond to treatment, as in the case of Dorothy above. At an individual patient level, this can lead to increased morbidity and, in severe cases, an increased risk of mortality. Dorothy could suffer additional discomfort whilst waiting for the new antibacterial drug to take effect, or, if severe, the untreated infection could develop into life-threatening sepsis. However, antimicrobial resistance has a wider impact on healthcare systems and society, and some examples of this are given below.

If the usual first line treatment for an infection is ineffective, an alternative drug will be required. This alternative may be less effective, have more adverse effects and be more costly (i.e. be less cost effective). Prolonged hospital inpatient stay due to ongoing infections, or increased numbers of admissions to allow administration of more complex antimicrobial treatment regimens, could also result in increased costs to the health system. As healthcare resources are not infinite, increased spending on antimicrobial medicines could impact services for patients with other conditions.

Many of the interventions made in healthcare might not be possible if there were a risk of untreatable infections caused by micro-organisms. For example, transplant operations requiring subsequent immunosuppressant therapy, chemotherapy for the treatment of cancer, and immune modulating treatments, such as those for rheumatoid arthritis and other inflammatory conditions, all impact a patient's immune response, increasing the chance of infection. If any resulting infection were unresponsive to antimicrobial treatment, the risk of mortality could outweigh the benefit of the intervention, making it unjustifiable. As seen during the COVID-19 outbreak, a severe viral infection can impact access to healthcare services more broadly, with even routine consultations cancelled. Any impact of this on disease outcomes and associated quality of life in the longer-term will become apparent over time.

Another potential implication of treatment-resistant infection, is the need to restrict movement of people and animals. Whilst IT solutions (such as video conferencing) can mitigate some of the implications of travel restrictions in relation to people, infections in animals have the potential to disrupt food chains.

Managing antimicrobial resistance

Limiting the development of antimicrobial resistance should be a consideration for healthcare professionals (HCPs) whatever their role and area of practice. For prescribers this might include reducing inappropriate antimicrobial usage and adhering to local advice regarding choice of antimicrobial drug. However, all HCPs can play a part in educating patients about the consequences of antimicrobial use, such as the importance of not requesting antibacterial drugs for self-limiting viral infections.

The report *Reframing resistance: How to communicate about antimicrobial resistance effectively* (Wellcome Trust, 2020) identified that the public had limited understanding of what is meant by antimicrobial resistance, and its consequences. The report identifies five principles of clearer communication that could help to address this. These include explaining the impact that antimicrobial resistance can have on the management of other illnesses such as cancer (as noted above), and the use of simple language to explain that antimicrobials are no longer working. The third principle aims to help patients see the personal effect of resistance, in particular, by explaining that it is not the person that becomes resistant but the micro-organism and as a result, anyone can be affected. Explaining that the impact of antimicrobial resistance is being seen at the present time and that things can be done to address the problem are the final principles.

At an organisational level, mechanisms to address resistance are termed antimicrobial stewardship, and this is discussed briefly below.

Antimicrobial stewardship

NICE guideline NG15 defines antimicrobial stewardship as 'an organisational or healthcare-system-wide approach to promoting and monitoring judicious use of antimicrobials to preserve their future effectiveness' (NICE, 2015). A number of recommendations for stewardship programmes and interventions are made. These include having mechanisms for the monitoring of antimicrobial usage and microbial resistance patterns and establishing teams to support prescribing through educational initiatives and medicine formulary guidance. When managing antimicrobial medicines, ensure that you are familiar with any available local guidance, with particular focus on treatment duration, dose and route of administration.

Environmental impact of medicines use

With growing concern over the environmental implications of human activity and global warming, the contribution to environmental damage made by medicines and healthcare activity has come into focus. Medicines and medicines management can have both direct and indirect effects on the environment, and some of these are considered briefly below.

Direct effects of medicines

Medicines and medical devices can have polluting effects on the air and water in our ecosystems, with implications for global warming and wildlife. Anaesthetic gases are typically vented to the atmosphere and have significant greenhouse effects (especially desflurane and nitrous oxide). Reducing waste may help to reduce the impact. Medical devices, such as pressurised metered dose aerosol inhalers, also directly contribute to greenhouse gas emissions. Switching patients to low-carbon-footprint inhalers (such as dry-powder devices), where appropriate, may be one way to address some of this burden. However, effective disease management through patient education could also help to reduce the need for bronchodilator therapy. More broadly, strategies to reduce air pollution could also help to reduce the incidence of respiratory and other diseases, reducing the need for these medicines.

Medicines may access water systems though elimination in faeces and urine (of both humans and animals), or by patients disposing of medicines inappropriately by flushing them in toilets. Sewage treatment is typically not designed to remove pharmaceuticals, which may therefore be discharged into rivers and other waterways. Drugs such as steroid hormones (e.g. oral contraceptives) and diclofenac have been shown to have a detrimental effect on fish, whilst the presence of antimicrobials may contribute to resistance. Although the scale of this pollution and effect on wildlife is difficult to quantify, the continued increase in medicines usage would suggest that any effect is only likely to increase over time. The European Medicines Agency has produced guidelines for the evaluation of environmental risk of medicines, which include an assessment of the effect on surface water.

Indirect effects of medicines

In addition to the direct polluting effects of medicines themselves, the way in which medicines are managed can also contribute to their environmental impact. Adverse drug reactions (ADRs) can lead to hospital admission, and the associated additional patient journeys may contribute to increased carbon emissions. As noted above, wastage may lead to inappropriate disposal of unwanted medicines with direct polluting effects. However, the manufacturing of medicines contributes to greenhouse emissions, and producing medicines that remain unused is associated with an environmental impact with no patient benefit. Medicine formulation may also have an impact with sterilisation of drugs intended for intravenous administration resulting in an increased carbon footprint. Aligned with this is the disposal of associated waste such as administration devices and packaging. With improved medicines management and advice to patients, it may be possible to reduce the number of ADRs and reduce reliance on medicines leading to reduced wastage.

Chapter summary

This chapter has explored some of the ways in which medicines can impact not only on the individual patient, but on society more widely. Although some of the adverse consequences of medicines use are seen at a societal level, principles of good medicines and disease management applied to the individual patient can help to address this. Educating patients on the value of vaccination and disease prevention, and the appropriate use (and risks associated with overuse) of medicines, is a key element of health promotion, and something that all healthcare professionals can contribute to.

Further reading

Public Health England (2021) Honest information about drugs: FRANK. www.talktofrank.com/

Provides information relating to substance use.

National Institute for Health and Care Excellence (2015) NG15 Antimicrobial stewardship: systems and processes for effective antimicrobial medicine use. Available at: www.nice.org. uk/guidance/conditions-and-diseases/infections/antimicrobial-stewardship. Accessed September 2021.

Provides guidance on antimicrobial stewardship.

Wellcome Trust (2020) *Reframing resistance: How to communicate about antimicrobial resistance effectively.* Available at: https://cms.wellcome.org/sites/default/files/2020-11/reframing-resistance-report.pdf. Accessed September 2021.

Provides recommendations for explaining antimicrobial resistance to patients.

World Health Organisation Fact Sheets (2020) Antimicrobial resistance. Available at: www.who. int/news-room/fact-sheets/detail/antimicrobial-resistance. Accessed September 2021.

Provides an overview of antimicrobial resistance, and management initiatives.

Chapter 8   Evidence-based medicines management

NMC Future Nurse: Standards of Proficiency for Registered Nurses

This chapter will address the following platforms and proficiencies:

Platform 1: Being an accountable professional

At the point of registration, the registered nurse will be able to:

1.7   demonstrate an understanding of research methods, ethics and governance in order to critically analyse, safely use, share and apply research findings to promote and inform best nursing practice.

1.8   demonstrate the knowledge, skills and ability to think critically when applying evidence and drawing on experience to make evidence-informed decisions in all situations.

1.20 safely demonstrate evidence-based practice in all skills and procedures stated in Annexes A and B.

Chapter aims

By the end of this chapter you should be able to:

1.   Consider some of the factors that affect the reliability of medicines-related information.
2.   Describe some of the study designs commonly used to evaluate the effects of medicines.
3.   Consider ways in which information derived from medicines research can be explained to patients.

Introduction

The information about medicines that you encounter in your practice will come from a variety of different sources. To be able to evaluate its usefulness, you will need to consider where the information has come from, what evidence it is based upon, and how it relates to your practice. If you judge it to be of value, you will then need to explain to your patients what it means, and encourage them to adopt it as part of the management of their condition. The Nursing and Midwifery Code (2018a) indicates that you should practise in line with the best available evidence, and that any advice you provide should be evidence-based. As with many aspects of medicines management, your ability to achieve this effectively will develop with experience; however, this chapter will give you an introduction to some of the things to consider.

Reliability of information

Case study

Scenario 1

Two weeks after starting your first placement as a student nurse, you visit your grandmother at her home. It is the first time that she has seen you since you started your training, and she is very excited to have a healthcare professional as a member of the family. She shows you a newspaper article that she has read, which suggests that eating a particular fruit can help with symptoms of arthritis. She asks whether you think eating this fruit instead of taking her prescribed medicines would be the best way for her to manage her arthritis.

Scenario 2

Whilst working on a ward, a pharmaceutical company sales representative gives a presentation to you and the rest of the multidisciplinary team about the company's new medicine for type 2 diabetes called Ionidestin. The presentation concludes that Ionidestin is better than other existing treatments, and the representative gives you a leaflet with some further information.

Activity 8.1   Reflection

Reflect on the scenarios presented in the above case study box, and answer the following questions:

1.   How would you respond to your grandmother's request for advice?
2.   What could affect the reliability of the information provided in the sales representative's presentation and leaflet?

An outline answer is given at the end of this chapter, and the text below also considers some of the issues raised.

The way in which information about medicines is presented can be influenced by a number of different factors. In both scenarios, you can see two different examples of how the author of the information might wish to present a particular point of view.

Many of your patients will read newspaper articles about their conditions and the medicines used to treat them. As a healthcare professional, you may be seen by your patients as an expert who can offer an opinion on the article, and any recommendations made. Remember that the aim of newspaper editors is to sell papers (or increase views on their website), and an eye-catching headline and the promise of a cure for a difficult-to-manage, painful condition is likely to increase sales. The article will probably have few specific details relating to the evidence in support of the particular fruit, without which it will be difficult to provide any definitive advice. Where possible, try to find the original source of the information, find out how the conclusion was reached, and evaluate the reliability of the headline (for more information on evaluating studies see below). Keep in mind that although you might not be a qualified nurse yet, patients and friends may see you as a healthcare professional who can provide reliable advice. You should ensure that the advice you give is correct or explain that you would have to find more information before you can give an opinion. Even if the information in the article is based upon good evidence, stopping a medicine and relying upon a particular food to manage an illness, without first seeking medical advice, may result in the return of symptoms and serious complications.

Whilst newspaper editors are trying to sell newspapers, pharmaceutical companies are trying to sell medicines (or at least encourage their prescribing). Although based upon clinical studies, the information provided by company representatives is likely to focus on the most positive aspects of the medicine and therefore be subject to a degree of bias. Once again, reading and evaluating the original source of the evidence that is summarised in a promotional presentation or leaflet will help to give a more balanced perspective of the effects of the drug.

Many patients will access information about their health and medicines using the internet. This can be a valuable and easily accessible source; however, the reliability of some of the information may be questionable. As with newspaper headlines, the original basis for statements that are made may not be clear, whilst in some cases, websites may actively promote misleading or malicious information to promote a particular viewpoint. Being able to identify and direct patients to reliable sources is important, and in the UK, the NHS website (www.nhs.uk) is a useful starting point.

Analysing and evaluating publications that provide evidence, and applying it to the management of a patient's medicines, forms the basis of practising 'evidence-based medicine'. The next part of this chapter will consider some of the different types of publications that provide evidence, and how you can start to evaluate them.

Medicines outcome studies – methodological design

This section considers some of the different approaches used to assess the effects of medicines, what they can tell us, and how they can be used to inform practice.

Activity 8.2   Critical thinking

During your training, you are looking after Phil, a 26-year-old man, who uses the recreational drug Spice (a synthetic version of cannabis). Phil is experiencing psychotic symptoms including hearing voices (hallucinations) and ideas that his neighbour is spying on him (delusions). You wonder whether this might be related to his use of Spice.

What research methodologies could you use to investigate a possible link between Spice use and psychotic symptoms?

As this activity is based on your own critical thinking, no outline answer is given at the end of this chapter. However, the text below explores some of the possible approaches that you could take.

Articles describing the effects of medicines that are published in medical and scientific journals can take a variety of forms. These range from large studies of many thousands of people, to reports describing an individual patient. Some study designs are seen to have greater value and be more important than others. The value attributed to the different forms of evidence (study designs or methods) used in these publications is sometimes referred to as the hierarchy of evidence. However, it could be argued that this is an oversimplification, as the different study designs all have their own advantages and limitations, and the findings should be considered with these in mind. Furthermore, the results of a poorly designed 'high-value' study may be of no greater use than those of a perceived 'low-value' study.

Case reports and case series

Perhaps the most straightforward type of article involves describing what has happened to a single patient or a small group of patients, known as a case report or case series respectively. In Activity 8.2, you could write a description of what you have noticed in the case of Phil, explaining how he uses Spice and has presented with symptoms of psychosis. Searching for other case studies describing the same effect would support your theory. Evidence derived from case studies or case series is considered low-value literature. This is because the number of patients included is small, and it is therefore difficult to know whether the effects that have been seen will apply to the wider population. Will everyone who uses Spice experience psychotic symptoms, or is it just Phil?

Finding some more Spice users and noting whether they have experienced psychosis will give a better picture and could form the basis of a 'case series'. However, even including ten people in a case series might represent a small proportion of the overall number of users and may not give the true picture. However, case reports and case series can offer a detailed account of what a patient or service user experienced and how they were managed, which may help to inform other clinicians when faced with a similar situation.

Randomised controlled trials (RCTs)

The randomised controlled trial (RCT) is often described as the 'Gold standard' approach to evaluate the effect of an intervention in medical literature. The aim of an RCT is to determine a causative link between an intervention (e.g. a medicine) and an outcome, by excluding other factors that may have influenced that outcome. The typical approach to an RCT of a medicine is to recruit a number of people with a given illness (the participants or sample), divide them into two or more groups and randomly assign them to treatment with the medicine of interest (the intervention), or to treatment with a different medicine or standard care (the comparator or control). The outcomes of the two groups (intervention and comparator) are then compared using a statistical approach to see whether they are different. In addition to being randomised and controlled, the trial may be 'blinded', where either the participants or study investigators, or both, do not know who receives which treatment. Alternatively, it may be 'unblinded' or 'open label', where the treatment that participants receive is known to the investigators and participants themselves.

The strength of an RCT is the method of recruiting participants who only have specific characteristics, and then randomly assigning treatment. Both of these elements help to reduce bias and to ensure that the result obtained is only due to the effect of the intervention, rather than other factors. However, whilst the RCT design is rigorous, it is expensive, and not always practical. If you wanted to investigate whether use of Spice was associated with psychotic symptoms, would it be ethical to recruit a group of people, give half of them Spice, and half of them a comparator, and see which group experienced more symptoms? You might find it difficult to recruit participants to a study like this! Another widely discussed limitation of RCTs is the nature of the participants. To minimise bias, RCTs have strict criteria that determine who can be included. This means that a typical patient that you might see in practice would not meet the entry criteria, and, as a result, the findings of the study might not be applicable to them. As a result, RCTs are not always 'generalisable' to the wider patient population. We have briefly discussed the exclusion of children and older adults from RCTs in previous chapters.

Observational studies

A different approach to evaluating the impact of an intervention is to use an 'observational' design. Observational studies involve identifying groups of people with certain characteristics of interest and looking to see if there are differences between them.

For example, you could identify a group of Spice users, see how many experienced psychotic symptoms over a period of time, and compare this to the development of psychotic symptoms in a group of non-Spice users. Alternatively, you could identify a group of people with psychotic symptoms, see how many use Spice, and compare them with a group of people without psychotic symptoms who use Spice. Because these study designs would not involve actively giving Spice to a group of participants, you are simply observing effects (hence 'observational studies'). This approach can help to overcome some of the potential ethical and recruitment barriers to an RCT. However, it is difficult to establish a causative link between the two factors (in this case Spice use and psychotic symptoms). This is because it is more difficult to ensure that the participants in each of the groups are the same, and that they don't have any characteristics that would bias the outcome. For example, your group of Spice users might be more likely to have been diagnosed with schizophrenia, and therefore be more likely to suffer from hallucinations and delusions as a result of their illness rather than their Spice use.

Meta-analysis

Meta-analysis is a statistical approach to combining the findings of several individual studies to give a more complete picture of the published literature. For example, there may be four studies linking Spice to psychotic symptoms, and one that suggests no link. If you combined all of the findings together, what would they tell you? The advantage of meta-analysis is that by combining data you can include information from a much larger number of participants. This makes it more likely that the findings are a correct estimate of what is happening in the whole population. If you think back to Phil as a single case, you cannot be certain that his psychotic symptoms after using Spice would be replicated in a wider population. If you combine the findings of five RCTs with a total of 3,500 participants, you can be a little more certain that the resulting outcome is the true answer to your question. Meta-analysis is often seen as the most valued evidence source due to this ability to include large participant numbers. However, like any study, if a meta-analysis is poorly designed, or the individual studies included in it are poorly designed, the results are less likely to be reliable.

Other study types

Although the study types listed above are probably the most encountered, you may see studies with other methods in the published literature. As noted above, a limitation of RCTs is that the findings may not apply to patients seen in day to day practice. To overcome this, 'naturalistic' studies report the effectiveness of medicines based upon observation of patient outcome in clinical practice. These studies usually lack comparator groups but are representative of real world experience of medicine use. Bridging the gap between naturalistic studies and RCTs, so-called 'pragmatic' trials, combine some of the rigour of RCTs, whilst using a more meaningful patient population. These studies are not usually blinded, so investigators and participants know which treatment they are receiving, which may introduce bias. Examples include the Clinical Antipsychotic Trials of Intervention Effectiveness (CATIE) study in schizophrenia (Lieberman et al., 2005), the SANAD study in epilepsy (Marson et al., 2007a, 2007b), and the Salford Lung study in respiratory conditions (New et al., 2014).

Audit and research

When working in a healthcare setting, you are likely to encounter audit, as a way of measuring the quality of a service. There are several differences between audit and research, including what they are intended to achieve, and how they are conducted. Table 8.1 illustrates some of the key differences.

Audit	Research
Systematically reviews an approach to care or treatment.	An investigation that will lead to the development of new knowledge, or increase the sum of existing knowledge.
Measures against a standard or benchmark.	Usually involves testing a hypothesis or idea.
Does not involve experiments or application of experimental methods.	Often involves experiments and in the case of medicines, experiments on human participants.
Does not evaluate the effectiveness of new interventions or treatments.	Used to evaluate the effectiveness of new interventions or treatments.
Does not involve changing a patient's treatment.	Often involves a change in treatment and disruption of the participant's regular intervention.
Does not involve randomisation.	May involve randomisation.

Table 8.1 Examples of differences between the Audit and Research.

Health technology appraisal

Although not a specific study design as such, Health Technology Appraisal (HTA) is an important aspect of medicines management and resource allocation. Funding for healthcare is limited, whether the system is based upon public or private money. It is therefore important to determine which medicines represent good value for money (and should be funded), and those that do not. HTA explores the benefits of a medicine compared to its cost (a cost-effectiveness analysis) and helps to ensure equity of access to cost-effective medicines across different therapeutic areas.

In HTA, evidence of a medicine's benefit is typically derived from RCT data, using a patient's quality and duration of life during treatment as the outcome measure. The cost of treatment includes the purchase cost of the medicine, as well as associated costs such as administration, managing adverse effects, healthcare professional intervention and any other relevant factors. A new medicine can then be compared to existing treatment to determine whether it is more or less effective and more or less costly. In the UK, this process is managed by the National Institute for Health and Care Excellence (NICE), the All Wales Medicines Strategy Group (AWMSG) and the Scottish Medicines Consortium (SMC). If the new medicine is judged to offer sufficient value at an acceptable cost, it will subsequently be funded by the National Health Service (NHS).

Evaluating studies

Case study

After hearing the pharmaceutical company sales representative's presentation on Ionidestin, you decide to do some research into this new drug. You find two published research papers, which are summarised below.

Paper 1:

An open label, randomised controlled trial, of 80 participants with type 2 diabetes, conducted in Brazil. Participants were randomly assigned by the study authors to receive Ionidestin or inactive placebo for 12 weeks. Participants were assessed at the start of treatment and at the end of treatment by the study authors. The primary outcome was change in HbA_{1c} level (an indicator of blood glucose level). Participants treated with Ionidestin had a statistically significantly greater reduction in HbA_{1c} (from 6.8 per cent to 4.9 per cent) than those treated with placebo ($p<0.01$).

Paper 2:

A double-blind, randomised controlled trial, of 3,600 participants with type 2 diabetes that hadn't responded well to previous treatment, conducted in the UK. Participants were randomly assigned (using a computer algorithm), to receive Ionidestin or inactive placebo added to their usual treatment for 52 weeks. Participants were assessed at the start of treatment, at monthly intervals and at the end of treatment by independent clinical researchers. The primary outcome was reduction in all-cause mortality, the secondary outcome was change in HbA_{1c} level. Participants treated with Ionidestin had a reduced incidence of mortality of 5 per cent compared with placebo ($p<0.05$), and a statistically significantly greater reduction in HbA_{1c} (from 7.1 per cent to 6.0 per cent) than those treated with placebo ($p<0.05$). The most common adverse effects were nausea, rash, and urinary tract infection, which occurred in 9 per cent of patients.

Activity 8.3   Critical thinking

Review the above case study. How would you evaluate the significance of these two papers?

An outline answer is given at the end of this chapter, and the text below considers some of the issues raised.

Reading and evaluating published literature is an important skill that will help you to identify whether the findings of a particular study can help in the management of your patients. At first glance, reading a published paper can seem a daunting prospect, and it is easy to simply focus on the abstract (summary of key points) without considering the detail of how the study was conducted. However, a review of the whole paper is important, as it can help to establish whether the study is relevant to your practice.

Published papers are usually divided into four sections, an introduction (explaining why the study is needed and what question it aims to answer), the methods (explaining what was done to answer the question), the results (explaining what the findings were) and the discussion (explaining what the findings mean). Before looking at the specific methods used, you should try to identify the question that the study is trying to answer. When looking at the methods, three key pieces of information to consider are the participants, the intervention and comparator, and the outcome measure. The sections below explore how these might affect the interpretation of the findings in the context of the two papers described briefly in the earlier case study.

Participants

The nature of, and way in which, participants are included in a study can have a significant impact on the interpretation of the findings. In the earlier case study, Paper 1 had a much smaller number of participants than Paper 2. As mentioned earlier in this chapter, the smaller the number of participants, the harder it is to draw conclusions about how the results might apply to a wider population.

The demographics of the participants also appear to be different in the two papers. Paper 1 was conducted in Brazil and Paper 2 in the UK. If you are working in the UK, Paper 2 is probably going to be more applicable to your practice, as there may be genetic or cultural differences that might influence the treatment outcome (and the opposite might be true if you were working in Brazil). Another difference in the studies was the nature of the disease being treated. Paper 2 included participants whose illness had not responded well to treatment, whereas Paper 1 did not specify a particular group. The characteristics of the participants of a study will be determined by the inclusion and exclusion criteria. These criteria might outline the age range, previous treatment and medical co-morbidities (as well as other factors) of participants. If these are not representative of the patients that you see, the study may have less relevance to your practice. It could also explain any differences in outcome. Ionidestin appeared to have a bigger effect on HbA_{1c} in Paper 1, however, the participants in Paper 2 had diabetes that hadn't responded well to previous treatment and might therefore be expected to show a smaller response.

Intervention and comparator

The method for allocating treatment can affect the outcome of a study. Although both studies were randomised, in Paper 1, allocation was managed directly by the investigators. This could lead to bias if the investigators put participants who they felt would respond better onto the active treatment. Using a computer algorithm or similar approach can help to overcome this limitation. The method used for randomisation should be reported in the methods section of a published paper. Blinding of the study is also designed to reduce possible bias. If the participants and investigators are unaware of who receives which treatment, there is less chance that this will influence the outcome. In the earlier case study, Paper 2 was double-blind (participants and investigators would not know which treatment was given), and therefore less likely to be susceptible to bias than Paper 1, which was open label (and where the treatment received would be known).

When considering the treatments used in a study, identify whether there is a comparator, and if so, what it is. In the earlier case study, Paper 1 used an inactive placebo comparator. Such studies present an ethical challenge, as some of the participants will not receive treatment for their disorder. In Paper 2, Ionidestin or placebo were added to participants' usual treatment, so even those in the placebo group received some form of active treatment. Another option is to compare the new drug to an existing, active treatment. You should consider whether the active treatment is part of the usual treatment for the disease in your healthcare system to judge the relevance to your practice. The choice of active comparator can also affect the study outcome. A comparator with unpleasant adverse effects could lead to more participants dropping out of the trial and an apparent advantage for the new medicine. If an active comparator is associated with a particular adverse effect, it may also affect the blinding of the study. If a patient experiences the adverse effect, the investigator will know which treatment was given, which might bias the outcome.

Outcome

The choice of outcome measure can have a significant impact on the interpretation of a study, and its relevance to practice. Paper 1 in the earlier case study used HbA_{1c} as the outcome measure. This indicates how good a patient's glucose control has been and is therefore relevant to diabetes. However, it does not really give an indication of whether the patients' overall health state was improved by the treatment. Using a measure such as mortality or stroke may provide a more valuable indication of treatment effect. The duration of each study was also different, with Paper 1 reporting a 12-week study, and Paper 2 a 52-week study. If the disease being investigated is a chronic illness, assessing the effects of the treatment over a 12-week period may be less relevant than a longer-term study.

Drug treatment trials are generally 'quantitative' studies (i.e. they generate numerical data). The data is analysed using statistics, to determine whether there are differences between the effects of the treatment under investigation and any comparator. A variety of statistical methods can be used, and an explanation of these is beyond the scope of this book. However, you should be able to identify some of the terminology used, such as 'statistically significant difference', and 'p value'. A statistically significant difference indicates that there is a difference between two sets of data. This could be the difference between the outcomes of the treatment group and the comparator group, or perhaps the incidence of certain adverse effects associated with each treatment. The p value gives an indication that findings are statistically significantly different. If a quoted p value is less than 0.05 ($p<0.05$), this generally indicates a statistically significant difference, with smaller p values, indicating stronger evidence to support that difference. In Paper 1 and Paper 2, the p values for reduction in HbA_{1c} with Ionidestin compared with placebo were <0.01 and <0.05 respectively, suggesting that Paper 1 had stronger evidence of an effect than Paper 2. It is important to note that although data from a study might indicate a statistically significant difference in effect between two treatments, it does not necessarily mean that there is a clinically significant difference in effect. This is a matter for clinical judgement.

Applying evidence to practice

Activity 8.4   Critical thinking

You are looking after Asim, a 47-year-old man with type 2 diabetes. His doctor has recommended that he takes Ionidestin in addition to his regular metformin to improve management of his diabetes. Asim asks you about the benefits and side effects of Ionidestin.

What would you tell him based on the findings of Paper 2 described in the earlier case study?

As this activity is based on your own critical thinking, no outline answer is given at the end of this chapter, however the text below explores some factors to consider.

The ability to explain information to patients is an important skill for all healthcare professionals. Patients should have access to reliable, up-to-date information to enable them to make informed decisions regarding their treatment. The level of detail needed when discussing different options will vary from person to person and should be tailored to the individual. Similarly, the degree to which different patients wish to engage in the decision-making process will vary. Some patients will be more familiar with a paternalistic approach, and less confident in expressing their views. A shared decision-making approach should nevertheless be encouraged, with consideration of how best to engage different individuals.

Key aspects to discuss with patients are the benefits and the risks associated with a treatment. Clear communication is important, and some of the approaches discussed in Chapter 6 are applicable here. Find out what the patient knows, and what they want to know about the treatment options they are considering. Be aware of the need for a translator, or the use of non-verbal communication aids, use plain language, and check that the patient understands the information.

A number of decision aids are available to support patients in the management of their conditions. These help to illustrate the benefits and risks of a particular strategy, compared to alternative treatments and also doing nothing. If a patient asks you about a new medicine, a specific decision aid may not be readily available. However, you may be able to adopt some of the approaches used. For example, when communicating risks and benefits, it may be more accessible to explain percentages as a number of people who are likely to experience the effect per population. Rather than telling Asim that 9 per cent of patients experience nausea, rash, and urinary tract infection with Ionidestin, you could express this as nine people in 100. The use of a diagram like the one in Figure 8.1 may help, with the sad faces in the panel on the left illustrating the proportion of patients likely to experience adverse effects, and the happy faces in the panel on the right the proportion likely to experience beneficial effects.

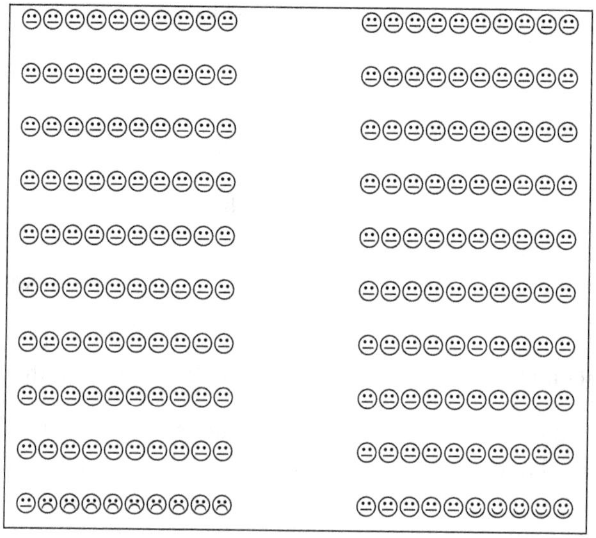

Figure 8.1 A 9% or 9 in 100 incidence of adverse effects illustrated by the sad faces in the panel on the left, and a 5% or 5 in 100 benefit illustrated by the happy faces in the panel on the right

It is important to note that when discussing risks and benefits, the nature of these is as important as the number of patients experiencing them. For example, although more people experience adverse effects of Ionidestin compared to the benefits, these are relatively minor (nausea, rash and urinary tract infection). Although the benefits are experienced by a smaller proportion of people than the adverse effects (5 per cent vs 9 per cent), five fewer people in 100 are less likely to die following 52 weeks of Ionidestin treatment (a very significant effect!). As well as explaining the absolute risk of an event (i.e. nine in 100 people experiencing an adverse effect), it may also help to explain how a medicine changes the risk of an event. For example, a drug may double the risk of a stroke. However, doubling the risk from one in ten to one in five may be more significant than doubling the risk from one in 10,000 to one in 5,000.

Chapter summary

To facilitate the use of safe, cost-effective medicines, it is important for practice to be based upon reliable, relevant and high-quality evidence. This chapter has introduced you to some of the types of evidence that you might encounter in your practice. Being able to interpret the findings of these and apply them to the management of your patients forms the basis of practising evidence-based medicine. This will help to ensure that your patients experience the best possible outcome from their treatment.

Activities: Brief outline answers

Activity 8.1 Reflection (page 140)

Whilst a healthy lifestyle and diet is an important aspect of disease management, medicines are a key part of managing symptoms and preventing future complications of many diseases. Stopping a medicine and relying upon a particular food to manage an illness, without first seeking medical advice, may result in the return of symptoms and serious complications.

Representatives from pharmaceutical companies are employed to promote the company's products and encourage their use. Information that they provide should be considered with this in mind. Leaflets and other material should include information based upon reliable sources such as published trials. However, the company may choose to highlight the more positive aspects of the trial in relation to their medicine, whilst ignoring some of the negative aspects (sometimes known as cherry-picking results).

Activity 8.3 Critical thinking (page 146)

Paper 1 describes a relatively small, open-label study, with allocation determined by the authors, therefore the findings may be more susceptible to bias and less reliable than those of the larger, double blind study described in paper 2. The study in paper 1 also had a shorter duration, only assessed HbA_{1c} rather than mortality, and did not appear to report any adverse effects, so it is less informative in relation to the possible outcomes of this patient group in practice.

Further reading

Freeman, ALJ (2019) How to communicate evidence to patients. *Drug and Therapeutics Bulletin* 57(8): 119–24.

Provides an overview of how to explain risks and benefits to patients.

Greenhalgh, T (2019) *How to read a paper: the basics of evidence based medicine and healthcare*, 6th Edition. John Wiley and Sons, Hoboken, NJ.

Provides an introduction to evidence-based medicine, and interpreting evidence.

References

American College of Obstetricians and Gynecologists' Committee on Practice Bulletins—Obstetrics (2019) ACOG Practice Bulletin No. 203: Chronic Hypertension in Pregnancy. *Obstet Gynecol.*, 133(1): e26-e50. doi: 10.1097/AOG.0000000000003020.

American Geriatrics Society (2019) Updated AGS Beers Criteria® for Potentially Inappropriate Medication Use in Older Adults. *J. Am Ger Society.* 67: 674–94.

British National Formulary. Medicines Guidance (2021). Controlled Drugs and drug dependence. Available at: https://bnf.nice.org.uk/guidance/controlled-drugs-and-drug-dependence.html

Edwards S and Axe S (2015). The 10 'R's of safe multidisciplinary drug administration. *Nurse Prescribing*, 13(8): 398–406.

Family Law Reform Act (1969) www.legislation.gov.uk/ukpga/1969/46/section/8

Gillick v West Norfolk and Wisbech AHA (1985) UKHL 7 (17 October 1985) www.bailii.org/uk/cases/UKHL/1985/7.html

Lieberman JA et al. (2005) Effectiveness of Antipsychotic Drugs in Patients with Chronic Schizophrenia. *New Eng J Medicine*, 353: 1209–23.

Marson AG et al. (2007a) The SANAD study of effectiveness of carbamazepine, gabapentin, lamotrigine, oxcarbazepine, or topiramate for treatment of partial epilepsy: An unblinded randomised controlled trial. *Lancet*, 369: 1000–15.

Marson AG et al. (2007b) The SANAD study of effectiveness of valproate, lamotrigine, or topiramate for generalised and unclassifiable epilepsy: An unblinded randomised controlled trial. *Lancet*, 369: 1016–26.

Mental Capacity Act (2005) Code of Practice. Available at: https://assets.publishing.service.gov.uk/government/uploads/system/uploads/attachment_data/file/921428/Mental-capacity-act-code-of-practice.pdf

Mental Health Act (1983) Code of Practice. Available at: https://assets.publishing.service.gov.uk/government/uploads/system/uploads/attachment_data/file/435512/MHA_Code_of_Practice.PDF

Mohsa RC and Greig NH (2017) Drug discovery and development: Role of basic biological research. *Alzheimers Dement (N Y)*, 3(4): 651–7. Available at: www.ncbi.nlm.nih.gov/pmc/articles/PMC5725284/

National Institute for Health and Care Excellence (NICE) (2014) SC1 Managing medicines in care homes. Available at: www.nice.org.uk/guidance/sc1

National Institute for Health and Care Excellence (NICE) (2015) NG15 Antimicrobial stewardship: Systems and processes for effective antimicrobial medicine use. Available at: www.nice.org.uk/guidance/conditions-and-diseases/infections/antimicrobial-stewardship. Accessed September 2021.

New JP et al. (2014) Obtaining real-world evidence: the Salford Lung Study. *Thorax* 69(12): 1152–4.

Nursing and Midwifery Council (2018a) The Code: Professional standards of practice and behaviour for nurses, midwives and nursing associates. London.

Nursing and Midwifery Council (2018b) Future Nurse: Standards of proficiency for registered nurses. London.

O'Mahony D et al. (2015) STOPP/START criteria for potentially inappropriate prescribing in older people: Version 2. *Age and Ageing*, 44: 213–18.

Pirmohamed M et al. (2004). Adverse drug reactions as cause of admission to hospital: prospective analysis of 18 820 patients. *Br. Med. J.*, 329: 15.

Plumpton CO et al. (2019) Cost-Effectiveness of panel tests for multiple pharmacogenes associated with adverse drug reactions: An evaluation framework. *Clinical Pharmacology and Therapeutics*, 105(6): 1429–38.

Quincy Bell and A -v- Tavistock and Portman NHS Trust and others (2020). www.judiciary.uk/judgments/r-on-the-application-of-quincy-bell-and-a-v-tavistock-and-portman-nhs-trust-and-others/

Royal Pharmaceutical Society (2018) Professional guidance on the safe and secure handling of medicines. Available at: www.rpharms.com/recognition/setting-professional-standards/safe-and-secure-handling-of-medicines/professional-guidance-on-the-safe-and-secure-handling-of-medicines?welcome=true

Royal Pharmaceutical Society (2019) Professional Guidance on the Administration of Medicines in Healthcare Settings.

Scottish Government Polypharmacy Model of Care Group (2018) Polypharmacy Guidance, Realistic Prescribing, 3rd Edition. Scottish Government. Available at: www.therapeutics.scot.nhs.uk/wp-content/uploads/2018/04/Polypharmacy-Guidance-2018.pdf. Accessed 11 January 2021.

Wellcome Trust (2020) Reframing resistance: How to communicate about antimicrobial resistance effectively. Available at: https://cms.wellcome.org/sites/default/files/2020-11/reframing-resistance-report.pdf. Accessed September 2021.

World Health Organisation (2017) Medication Without Harm: Global Patient Safety Challenge on Medication Safety. Geneva: World Health Organization. Licence: CC BY-NC-SA 3.0 IGO.

World Health Organisation (2019) *Medication Safety in Transitions of Care.* Geneva: World Health Organization; (WHO/UHC/SDS/2019.9). Licence: CC BY-NC-SA 3.0 IGO.

Wouters OJ, McKee M and Luyten J (2020) Estimated Research and Development Investment Needed to Bring a New Medicine to Market, 2009–2018. *JAMA*, 323(9): 844–53. doi: 10.1001/jama.2020.1166. https://jamanetwork.com/journals/jama/article-abstract/2762311

Index

Locators in *italics* refer to figures and those in **bold** to tables.

CPSIA information can be obtained
at www.ICGtesting.com
Printed in the USA
JSHW060022100423
40043JS00002B/84

9 781529 730814